# ADVANCES IN CLINICAL NEUROPHYSIOLOGY

Edited by **Ihsan M. Ajeena**

**Advances in Clinical Neurophysiology**
http://dx.doi.org/10.5772/3178
Edited by Ihsan M. Ajeena

**Contributors**

Hiromu Katsumata, Dongyu Wu, Ying Yuan, Pierre Rabischong, Yuko Urakami, Andreas A. Ioannides, George K. Kostopoulos, Fariba Eslamian, Mohammad Rahbar, Fernando Peña-Ortega, Ignacio Rodríguez-Carreño, Luis Gila-Useros, Armando Malanda-Trigueros, Štefania Rusnáková, Ivan Rektor, D. V. Moretti, G. B. Frisoni, G. Binetti, O. Zanetti

**Published by InTech**

Janeza Trdine 9, 51000 Rijeka, Croatia



**Publishing Process Manager** Vedran Greblo
**Technical Editor** InTech Prepress, Novi Sad
**Cover** InTech Design team

Additional hard copies can be obtained from orders@intechopen.com

Advances in Clinical Neurophysiology, Edited by Ihsan M. Ajeena
p. cm.
ISBN 978-953-51-0806-1

For EU product safety concerns:
IN TECH d.o.o., Prolaz Marije Krucifikse Kozulić 3, 51000 Rijeka, Croatia,
info@intechopen.com or visit our website at intechopen.com.

# Meet the editor

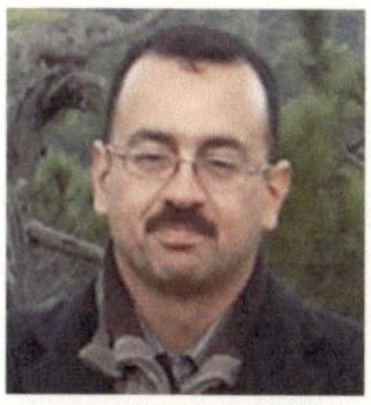

Ihsan Mohammad Abud Ajeena (MBChB, MSc, PhD Physiology (Neurophysiology)) is an Assistant Professor of Physiology at College of Medicine, University of Kufa, Iraq. He is the representative and general secretary of the Iraqi branch of the International Federation of Clinical Neurophysiology (IFCN). Dr. Ajeena has more than 10 years of experience in different disciplines of clinical neurophysiology. He has supervised many postgraduate students and has published many scientific articles in his field of research. He has also participated in many related national and international symposiums, conferences and workshops.

# Contents

**Preface IX**

Chapter 1 **The Examination of Cortical Dynamics for Perceptual-Motor Processes in Visually-Guided Cognitive/Motor Task Performances 1**
Hiromu Katsumata

Chapter 2 **Electroencephalography (EEG) and Unconsciousness 31**
Dongyu Wu and Ying Yuan

Chapter 3 **The Skin Neural Interface 55**
Pierre Rabischong

Chapter 4 **Sleep Spindles – As a Biomarker of Brain Function and Plasticity 73**
Yuko Urakami, Andreas A. Ioannides and George K. Kostopoulos

Chapter 5 **Neuromuscular Disorders in Critically-Ill Patients – Approaches to Electrophysiologic Changes in Critical Illness Neuropathy and Myopathy 109**
Fariba Eslamian and Mohammad Rahbar

Chapter 6 **Pacemaker Neurons and Neuronal Networks in Health and Disease 121**
Fernando Peña-Ortega

Chapter 7 **Motor Unit Action Potential Duration: Measurement and Significance 133**
Ignacio Rodríguez-Carreño, Luis Gila-Useros and Armando Malanda-Trigueros

Chapter 8 **The Neurocognitive Networks of the Executive Functions 161**
Štefania Rusnáková and Ivan Rektor

Chapter 9 **Mild Cognitive Impairment and Quantitative EEG Markers: Degenerative Versus Vascular Brain Damage 171**
D. V. Moretti, G. B. Frisoni, G. Binetti and O. Zanetti

# Preface

Clinical neurophysiology is a continuously growing branch of medical sciences that tends to link itself with unlimited number of other medical and surgical specialties. Recently, it is known that clinical neurophysiology is becoming increasingly important not only for the early diagnosis of some diseases but also because it can be applied within some surgical fields and within the intensive care units. Neurophysiology is also important for long term monitoring of some patients despite its role in curing many entities of diseases. It also has a role to monitor the progress of some diseases in response to different modalities of treatment.

The emergence of new diagnostic and therapeutic applications of this field necessitate that neurophysiologists master these medical arts and participate actively in them in order to consolidate and develop new concepts to meet the increasing demand of evidence-based medicine aiming to ameliorate human well being and eliminate patient suffering.

*Advances in Clinical Neurophysiology* is not simply a handbook of neurophysiology. I strongly encourage neurophysiologist and clinicians interested in this field to get this book as many advance techniques and findings in clinical neurophysiology are presented.

I am sincerely grateful to the brilliant, talented and experienced authors that participated in this edition and for their patience and kind compliance with my requests. My deep gratitude should be extended to the publishing managers and the publisher for their support and continuous commitment to complete this book.

Hoping to enlighten new neurophysiologic diagnostic and therapeutic ideas, I herby present this book to you, dear reader. I will be awaiting your kind scientific feedback because without constructive feedback we cannot improve ourselves.

**Ass. Prof. Dr. Ihsan M. Ajeena**
College of Medicine - University of Kufa
Iraq

Chapter 1

# The Examination of Cortical Dynamics for Perceptual-Motor Processes in Visually-Guided Cognitive/Motor Task Performances

Hiromu Katsumata

Additional information is available at the end of the chapter

http://dx.doi.org/10.5772/50263

## 1. Introduction

### 1.1. Importance of perceptual process for goal-directed movements

Goal directed movements are organized via perceptual information that is relevant to movement situation. Even in a simple movement of reaching out a glass on a table and grasping it, the configuration and orientation of hand and fingers should be organized with respect to the size, shape, and orientation of the glass. According to the study on prehensile movements, the size of aperture shaped by an index finger and a thumb to grasp an object was organized with respect to the size of the object such that the peak aperture was observed well before the hand reaches the object and the peak value was linearly scaled to the object's size (Jeannerod, 1981, 1984). When a mechanical perturbation was applied to an upper arm during a prehensile movement to assist or disturb the hand reaching an object, the well-coordinated reaching and grasping components was observed in terms of timing the grasping movement with respect to the moment of the hand reaching the object (Haggard & Wing, 1995). For pre-shaping the aperture and temporally organizing the reaching-grasping components, perceptual information about the object size and the time to the hand-object contact is crucial. Therefore, how perceptual process plays a role for organizing a movement and what/how perceptual information is utilized for the movement organization have been major issues in the study of motor control.

### 1.2. Two cortical pathways for visual information processing

According to the study on the cortical function for visual processing, there are two visual streams from the primary visual cortex to the posterior parietal cortex (the dorsal stream) and to the inferotemporal cortex (the ventral stream). Lesions to one of these visual pathways induce different types of perceptual-motor deficits. The lesions associated with the dorsal stream (e.g., the occipitoparietal region) induce the inability to shape the prehensile aperture for reaching and grasping an object properly but with no difficulty in visually discriminating one such object from another. Contrary to it, the lesions associated with the ventral stream (e.g., the ventrolateral region) leads to the reverse deficit (i.e., the inability to visually discriminate the object with the intact aperture control for grasping). Therefore, these findings have been regarded as the evidence of two visual processing pathways, one for visuomotor control via the dorsal stream, and the other for cognitive visual processing via the ventral stream (Goodale et al., 1994).

### 1.3. Cognitive aspect of perceptual-motor process for executing task performances

From a computational or information processing point of view (e.g., Schmidt & Lee, 1999), the cognitive process of recognizing the identity of an object to be grasped and planning how to produce a grasping movement with respect to the recognized object's shape, size, and orientation is central for organizing a prehensile movement. Such cognitive aspect of visual information processing for achieving perceptual-motor tasks with respect to a target object has been studied by an experimental paradigm using an target object, such as, the Ebbinghaus figure or Müller-Lyer figure that induces a visual illusion about the object size.

In this experimental paradigm, the following two perceptual-motor tasks have been used: 1) reaching out toward and grasping a visual object with an index-thumb pinch grip, and 2) assessing the size of the same visual object and indicating the estimated size by the same aperture as used to grasp the object. These two tasks share a qualitatively similar perceptual-motor process in terms of producing the same aperture configuration based on the same visual information about the target figure. However, the involvement of cognitive process (i.e., recognizing the target object, estimating its size, and deciding the grasping aperture size with respect to the perceived object size) seems to be different. In the size-estimation task, the production of the aperture configuration requires explicit identification of the size of the figure and the particular aperture size needs to be associated arbitrary with respect to the particular perceived size of the figure. In this sense, executing this task is cognitive process-oriented (Ranganathan & Carlton, 2007). As for the reaching-grasping task, the study on modeling a prehensile movement with nonlinear equations of motion, which include a perceptual variable as a parameter to modulate the dynamics of the movement, demonstrated the spatial and temporal characteristics of upper limb kinematics in the prehensile motion (Schöner, 1994; Zaal, 1998). This result supports the idea in the theoretical frameworks of the ecological perspective (Lee, 1980; Turvey & Kugler, 1984; Warren, 1990) and dynamical system account (e.g., Kelso, 1995; Schöner & Kelso, 1988) for motor coordination such that organizing a prehensile movement may not necessarily involve a cognitive process, such as the object identification and the arbitral object-aperture size association. From the above perspective, the perception of a target object and an action with respect to it are mutually dependent in the grasping task, whilst those in the size-estimation task are uncoupled and mediated via the cognitive process.

The original findings in the seminal studies using the paradigm were such that visual discrimination or perception about the object's size was susceptible to the illusory object, but the grasping aperture with respect to it was not (e.g., Aglioti et al., 1995; Haffenden & Goodale, 1998). An argument based on these findings has been such that cognitive perceptual processing and motor production process can be dissociable (Goodale & Milner, 1992) and the theoretical confrontation between the cognitive account for information processing in organizing a movement (e.g., Schmidt & Lee, 1999) and the ecological perspective for the perceptual-motor process (e.g., Lee, 1980; Turvey & Kugler, 1984; Warren, 1990) can be ascribed to these two visual streams (Tresilian, 1995). However, contradictory result has been reported such that the effect of the misperception about the object size was also observed in a prehensile movement (e.g., Franz, et al., 2000; Franz, et al., 2001). Other studies also found the susceptibility to the illusory object in a prehensile movement and suggested: the involvement of the ventral stream involved in a grasping motion with respect to a complex object (McIntosh, et al., 2004); the partial, not exclusive, dissociation between the two pathways (Ellis, et al., 1999); a multiple visuomotor process involving both pathways (Westwood, et al., 2000b); and the execution of prehensile movements by involving the ventral stream via the supplementary motor areas (Lee & van Donkelaar, 2002).

## 1.4. Examination of cortical activities in perceptual-motor performances

The above findings suggest that integrated function of cortical networks for executing the visuo-motor task needs to be considered for fully understanding the mechanism of the perceptual-motor process. From this view, the present study examines the cortical activation pattern during the reaching-grasping and the size-estimation performances. A particular focus for this investigation is on how cortical activities associated with the dorsal and ventral streams are involved in the perceptual-motor process for the task performances.

For this investigation, it is necessary to assess the effect of the perception of the target object size on the task execution. Therefore, the two task movements were produced with respect to a neutral object and an object inducing a size illusion (the Ebbinghaus figure). The illusion effect on the aperture configuration indicates that cognitive processing is involved in the task execution. In the case of the size-illusion effect observed in the size-matching performance but in the grasping, the observed cortical activities are interpreted in terms of the differences in association between cognitive processing and movement execution. If distinctive activation patterns between the two task performances are observed, it may be attributed to the difference in the perceptual-motor process associated with the involvement of cognitive processing. Conversely, if no difference in the cortical activity patterns between them, it may suggests some qualitative similarity in the cortical process between the different task executions.

On the other hand, the illusion effect on both of the tasks performances indicates that cognitive process is involved even in the reaching-grasping performance. In this case, the point of comparison in cortical activities between the two task conditions may not whether the dorsal and ventral streams are exclusively functioned, but how worked as an integrated cortical network. If difference in the pattern of cortical activities is observed, it reflects qualitative difference in the participation of cognitive process in the task movement execution.

### 1.5. Examination of the brain dynamics related to task execution

To investigate the cortical activity, electroencephalograph (EEG) during the task performance was analyzed in terms of frequency domain. Two different analyses, which potentially shed light on the different aspects of cortical activities, were conducted: the change of the EEG frequency power spectrum that was time-locked to the task event (Event-related spectral perturbation: Makeig, 1993; for review, Pfurtscheller et al., 1999a) and the coherence between EEGs of two electrodes (Event-related coherence: e.g., for review, Hummel & Gerloff, 2006; Schlögl & Supp, 2006; Pfurtscheller & Andrew, 1999).

Event-related spectral perturbation (ERSP) quantifies the degree to which the amplitude of a particular frequency band of ongoing EEG attenuates or enhances in response to a stimulus event, which is termed event-related desynchronization (ERD) or synchronization (ERS), respectively. ERD has been regarded as representing an activated cortical state with which the processing of sensory, motor, or cognitive information is enhanced and the excitability of cortical neurons is increased (Pfurtscheller, 2001; Steriade et al., 1991), whilst ERS has been thought that it reflects a deactivated cortical state with reduced information processing or none at all and decreased cortical excitability (Neuper & Pfurtscheller, 2001; Pfurtscheller, 1992). However, the knowledge about the ERS has been accumulated such that the meaning of ERS is more than the state of decreased cortical excitability. The inhibitory activity of ERS can play a functional role to accentuate a task-related information processing by inhibiting other cortical areas and/or to deactivate some cortical network depending on a task context/situation (Neuper & Pfurtscheller, 2001; Hummel et al., 2002, 2006; Suffczynski et al., 1999).

Coherence refers to correlation between two sets of time-series in frequency domain. Given a cross-spectral density matrix by two time series (i.e., EEG data from two electrodes), coherence is obtained by the ratio of cross-spectral to spectral of each time series, which indicates the degree of relative synchrony between the two time series, as shown below:

$$Coherence: C_{ij}(f) = \frac{|S_{ij}(f)|^2}{S_{ii}(f)S_{jj}(f)}$$

where $S_{ii}(f)$ and $S_{jj}(f)$ refers to frequency spectral of electrode $i$ and $j$ at frequency $f$, respectively, and $S_{ij}(f)$ refers to cross-spectral of electrode $i$ and $j$ at $f$. Higher coherence means higher degree of coupling between the two EEGs, which is interpreted as functional connectivity between two cortical sites. This idea of coherence has been extended for taking into consideration about the effect of temporal relationship between two time series to examine if one time series has influence on the other, and vice versa. This is termed directed coherence (Saito & Harashima, 1981; Kamitake, et al., 1984 cited in Wang & Takigawa, 1992). Analyzing the time series data with respect to a task event can reveal the change in the directed coherence over time with respect to the event (event-related directed coherence: EvDirCoh). By applying the EvDirCoh analysis to a set of EEG data over the cortex, functional connectivity or communication between different cortical sites and the direction of the communication for perceptual-motor process to execute a task performance can be investigated.

For these two analyses, the author and his colleagues analyzed ERSP in the reaching-grasping and the size-estimation performances (Katsumata, et al., 2009). Given the findings by the previous analysis that revealed the cortical activation pattern for the task execution, the present study conducts the EvDirCoh analysis for the data to investigate the cortical communication across different sites. Thereby, it is attempted to capture the brain dynamics characteristic to the perceptual-motor process for the task execution. In this chapter, experimental and analytical methodology for both of ERSP and EvDirCoh and those results are reported, and the dynamics of cortical activation is discussed in terms of the association of cognitive aspect with respect to the perceptual-motor process.

## 2. Methods

### 2.1. Participants

10 healthy participants volunteered for the experiment (seven males and three females with an average age of 29 ± 6.7 years). Their preferred hands for performing task movements were right hand and they were assessed as being right-handed by the Edinburgh inventory. All procedures were approved by an ethics committee. Each participant signed an informed consent form after the experimenter explained the purpose and procedure of the experiment.

### 2.2. Task and task conditions

Two types of perceptual-motor tasks were examined (Figure 1): (1) the participants reached out with their right hands to a target object displayed on the computer screen and touched it so as to grasp it with a pinch grip produced by the index finger-thumb aperture (*Grasping*) and (2) they produced the pinch grip as in *Grasping* task but without the reaching motion, so as to match the index-thumb aperture size with respect to the target object size (*Matching*).

Two different figures were used as the target objects: (1) a single circle with a diameter of 3 cm (*Neutral figure*) and (2) the *Ebbinghaus figure*, consisting of a center circle with a 3 cm diameter surrounded by five circles with 5 cm diameters. In *Matching*, the participants were instructed to estimate the size of the center circle and show it with the index finger-thumb aperture size. The aperture motion was the same as in *Grasping* but without reaching. The aperture size against the *Ebbinghaus figure* was produced the with respect to the center circle. Approximately one second after holding the aperture configuration, they terminated the task movement (Figure 2 for the time course of the task paradigm).

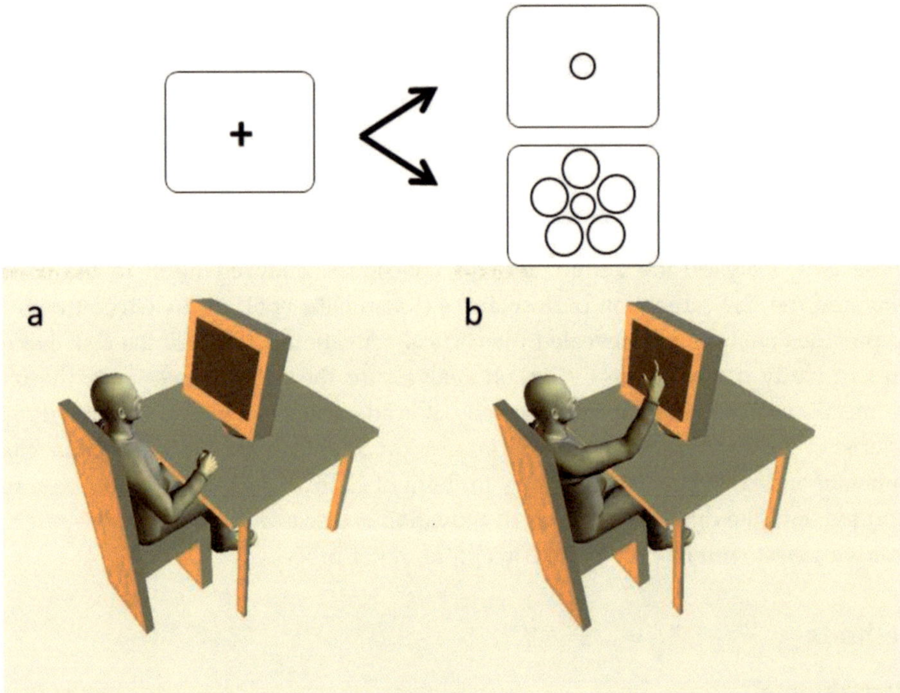


**Figure 1.** Schematic picture of the experiment task
(a) A starting posture and hand position before performing the task. (b) In Grasping, a participant reached out the target figure on the computer display and made a pinch-grasp without touching the display. In *Matching,* the same pinch-grip was produced with the starting posture. For the insets above, refer to the experimental procedure in the main text.

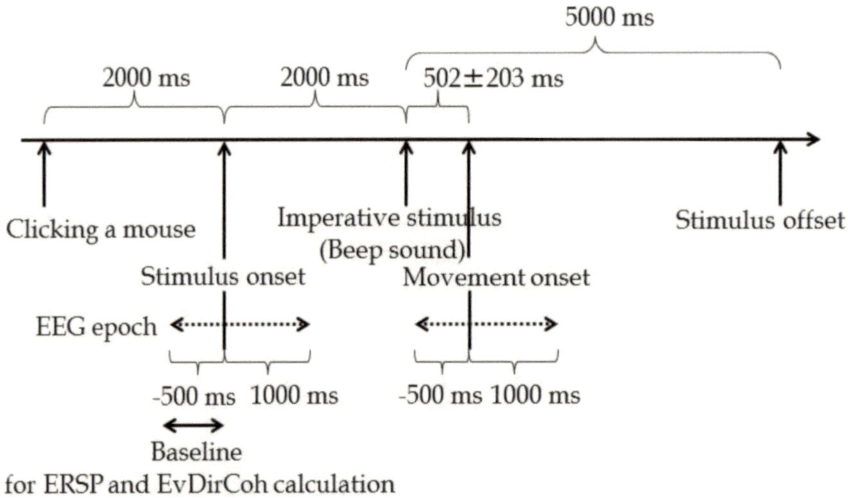


**Figure 2.** Time course of the task paradigm

## 2.3. Setup

The aperture movement was measured in terms of the angular excursion of the metacarpophalangeal joint by attaching a Goniometer (DKH, Tokyo, Japan) to the index finger. To this end, casts were attached to the proximal and distal interphalangeal joints of index finger and thumb. Thereby, the motions of these joints were constrained such that the aperture size was produced by only the movement of the index finger-metacarpophalangeal joint. This measure of the joint excursion was used to examine the grasping aperture. A 64-channel data collection system (ESI-64 Channel System, Neuroscan, Charlotte, NC) was used to collect Electroencephalogram (EEG). The visual display of the target figure, a beep sound to cue the participant to initiate the task movement, a trigger pulse to synchronize the Goniometer data with EEG data were operated by a data collection software (LabView, National Instruments, Austin, TX)

## 2.4. Procedure

Preliminary to the data collection, the effect of the Ebbinghaus figure for each participant was tested by the method of limit. By verbally judging the comparison between the size of a center circle of the Ebbinghaus figure with a comparison object of a single circle with different sizes, the perceptual threshold for detecting the size difference was examined (mean and standard deviation: 2.8±0.15 cm, as opposed to 3 cm of the center circle diameter of the Ebbinghaus figure). A t-test confirmed that the participants visually perceived the *Ebbinghaus figure* to be smaller than the comparison circle ($p < 0.01$).

The procedure of data collection was as follows (Figure 2). At the beginning of each trial, a "+" symbol was displayed at the center of the screen as a visual fixation point. After the participant clicked a computer mouse with their left hands, the fixation point disappeared. 2000 ms after the fixation offset, the target figure was shown at the center of the display. 2000 ms after the target onset, a beep sound was produced to cue the participants to initiate the task movements. 5000 ms after the auditory cue, the target figure disappeared, and it was enough time for the movement to be completed. Thereafter, the fixation point appeared for next trial. In instructing a task procedure to the participants, it was emphasized that the task was not for testing a reaction time nor a speed of task movement (The mean time of the movement initiation after the beep: 502±203 ms). The 80 trials of task movements for each condition were divided into two blocks consisting of 40 trials and performed in series. The order of *Grasping* and *Matching* was counterbalanced across the participants. The order of the figures across trials was randomized within each set of trials. They could take a few minutes break between blocks, and they could also take an inter-trial interval, during which they could blink. By these brakes, the participants could complete the whole set of trials without getting too fatigued. The whole data collection process lasted for approximately 90 minutes for each participant.

## 2.5. Data collection and reduction

The movement of index finger metacarpophalangeal joint was recorded (400Hz) by the Goniometer and a second order band-pass filter with a cutoff frequency of 5 Hz was used for smoothing the data. The angular velocity of the joint was obtained by numerical differentiation and smoothed by a second order band-pass filter (cutoff frequency of 5 Hz). EEG was collected from 64 scalp electrodes of the international 10-20 system referenced to the left earlobe (AC-mode, a sampling rate of 1000 Hz, a gain of 500, and a pass-band of 0.05-100 Hz). All electrodes were required a resistance of less than 2 Ω. To detect horizontal and lateral eye movements as well as blinks, electrooculography (EOG) of the right eye was collected. The data sets of EEG, joint movements, and auditory beeps were stored in the hard-drive of a desktop PC for off-line analysis. In the analysis, the EEG data was down-sampled to 300 Hz to conserve the memory of the PC and to save time consuming for calculating the coherence for each time-window within each frequency band. Failed trials due to initiating the movement before the auditory cue were eliminated from the analysis. The trials with an eye blink and noisy EEG data were also eliminated through visual inspection of EEG data profiles. EEG data was investigated with respect to the moments of the target onset and the initiation of the joint motion. To this end, EEG data sets for each trial were epoched from 500 ms before to 1000 ms after the target onset as well as after the initiation of the joint motion. Given the time from the movement onset to the maximum aperture of 626±198 msec, this time window was enough to cover the movement duration to produce the aperture configuration. For analysing EEG data with respect to specific frequency components, following frequency bands were used, delta: 0.5-4 Hz, theta: 4-8 Hz, alpha: 8-13 Hz, beta: 13-30 Hz, gamma: 30-45 Hz, and higher gamma: 45Hz-100Hz.

## 2.6. Analysis

### *2.6.1. Kinematics of task performances*

While reaching to grasp an object, the maximum aperture by the index finger and thumb is linearly related to the object's size (Jeannerod, 1981, 1984). Since this maximum preshape aperture is formed well before the hand has any contact with the object, this measure has been interpreted as reflecting the size estimate used in the perceptual-motor process in the prehensile activities. Based on this finding, the maximum aperture has been used as a dependent variable in many studies to investigate the influences of visual illusions on grasping (e.g., Haffenden & Goodale, 1998; Westwood,et al, 2000a; Franz et al., 2001). Because of this, the peak joint angle measured by the Goniometer was used as the measure of the maximum aperture for the prehensile movement. The time of the joint movement initiation was determined by the start of flexion movement of the metacarpophalangeal joint, at which the velocity of the joint kinematics started to show a positive value. This measure was used to epoch the EEG with respect to the onset of task movement.

### *2.6.2. Analysis of the event-related spectral perturbation*

The event-related spectral perturbation (ERSP) analysis was conducted by using a toolbox with graphic interface, EEGLAB, that is operated under the MATLAB environment (Delorme & Makeig, 2004). The epoched window of 1500 msec in a single trial was divided into brief subwindows of 214 msec with a sliding latency of 3.3 msec, corresponding to 98 %

overlapping between the successive subwindows. Wavelet analysis using sinusoidal transform was conducted for each of the subwindowed-epochs, and it obtained power spectrum estimates ranging from 0.59 Hz to 99.6 Hz with a frequency increment of 0.59 Hz. The power spectra over the sliding latency windows were computed for each trial, and normalized by subtracting baseline spectrum from each spectrum estimate. The baseline spectra were obtained by computing the mean spectra of the EEG data windowed for 500 msec before the moment of the target onset. Mean ERSP was obtained on each participant basis by computing the average of the baseline-normalized ERSP across all trials. To capture visually the global picture of ERSP, the grand average ERSP across the participants was plotted on the 3D time-frequency space (a spectrogram) on which the power spectrum of each frequency (in dB) at each sliding time-window was indicated by a colored surface.

The significance of increase/decrease in the power spectra with respect to the baseline spectra was examined for the mean ERSP in each time-frequency component of the spectrogram on each participant basis. To this end, non-parametric tests (a two-tailed Wilcoxon signed-rank test) was conducted with the null-hypothesis of no difference between the baseline spectra and spectra of each time-frequency components (i.e., ERSP value is zero) and the significant level of $p < .05$. This test was conducted for all of the time-frequency components. The difference in ERSP pattern between *Grasping* and *Matching* conditions was examined by the two-tailed Wilcoxon signed-rank test ($p < .05$) for each of time-frequency components. The results of z-values, which revealed the significant "*Grasping-Matching*" differences, for each time-frequency component, were plotted on a time-frequency plane. This gives the general view about the distribution of the significant ERS/ERD difference between the task conditions over the cortex.

In the previous study by the author and his colleagues (Katsumata et al., 2009), the ERSP analysis described above was conducted for 55 electrodes over the cortex with further analysis to summarize the characteristics of those ERSP profiles. For reporting the results in this chapter, ERSPs of the electrodes on the left-hemisphere were focused.

## 2.7. Analysis of event-related directed coherence

Event-related directed coherence (EvDirCoh) was calculated by the program operated under the MATLAB environment, which was developed by Takahasi, Baccalá and Sameshima (2008). For the calculation, the EEG time series were detrended before coherence calculation, Nuttall-Strand algorithm was used for estimating multivariate autoregressive models (MAR), and Akaike information criterion (AIC) was used for the criterion to choose the MAR order. The coherence was calculated with the time-window of 60ms with 30 ms increment, resulting in 15 time-windows from 500 ms to 1000 ms after the onset of target figure and task movement, and with respect to each of frequency bins. The time windows and frequency bins were set coarser than those used for the ERSP analyzes, since executing the program for calculating directed coherence was much more time consuming, given the number of electrode combinations for calculating the coherence. However, the preliminary analysis, for some of the data, using the finer time windows and frequency bins confirmed that this does not lose information about the global picture of coherence pattern over time and across frequencies.

Mean EvrDirCoh across trials within each participant was obtained for *Grasping* and *Matching* conditions respectively and subjected to a two-tailed Wilcoxon signed-rank test if the event-related coherence was significantly different from the baseline coherence ($p < .05$). This test was conducted for each of the time-frequency components. The baseline coherence was obtained by the mean coherence for the time window of 500 msec before the moment of the target onset. Only the EvrDirCohs, which were significantly higher than the baseline coherence, were subjected for reporting the results. A set of significant EvrDirCoh across all the time-windows and frequency bins were plotted on a time-frequency plane, which shows how coherence within a particular frequency band increased or decreased over time with respect to the onset of target figure and/or task movement (Figure 3).

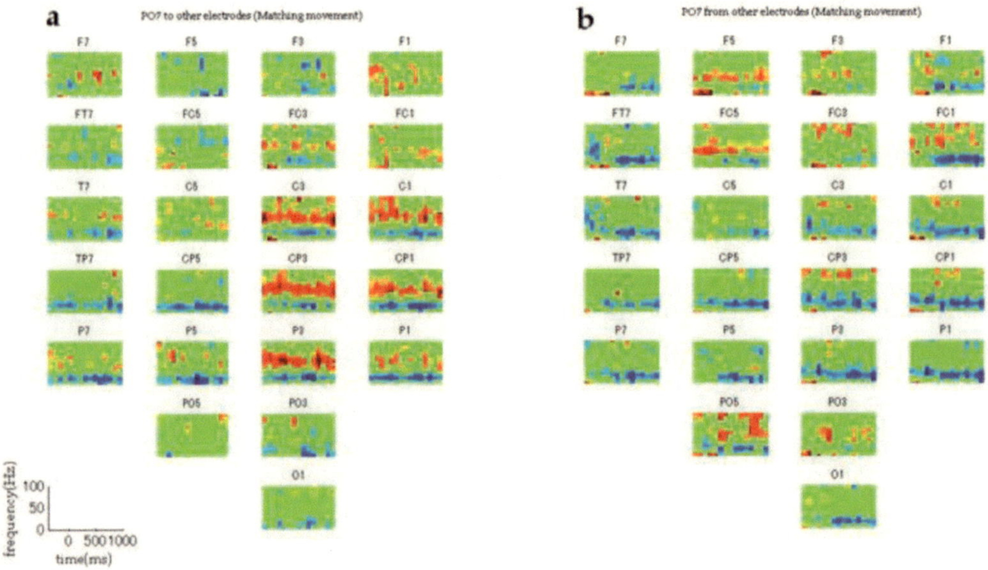


**Figure 3.** Time-frequency plot, Exemplary time-frequency plot of EvDirCoh from PO7 in *Matching* ,(a) EvDirCoh from PO7 to other electrode, and (b) to PO7 from other electrodes on the left-hemisphere. For each plot, EvDirCoh, which was significantly higher (red) and lower (blue) than the baseline coherence, and the non-significant time-frequency components (light green) were shown. Each electrode name was shown top of each plot.

Calculating the coherence of all the electrodes available was redundant. Even in the left-hemisphere, there were 24 electrodes leading to 23 time-frequency plots in one direction of EvDirCoh and another 23 plots for the other direction. Therefore, the present study focused on the electrodes in the left-hemisphere, which cover the cortical sites associated with the dorsal/ventral stream and visuomotor process in a hand movement against a visual target (O1, PO3, PO7, P3, P7, CP3, TP7, C3, T7, FC3, FT7, F3, and F7), but it still lead to 299 plots for coherence in the one direction and another 299 for the other direction. Since the primary aim of the study was to capture the global characteristics of EvDirCoh pattern over the cortex, it was attempted to summarize the results of the EvDirCoh plots in the following procedures.

### *2.7.1. Electrode combinations showing marked EvrDirCoh*

To capture what electrode combinations revealed marked EvrDirCoh, the rate of significant EvrDirCoh was calculated for each time-frequency plot. To this end, the number of time-frequency components on a time-frequency plane within a particular time-window, which showed the significant EvrDirCoh, was divided by the total number of time-frequency components within the corresponding time-window, and multiplied by 100 to show the result in percent. The ranges of time window were: (1) 500 ms from the target onset; (2) 500 ms before the onset of task movement to 100 ms after the onset; and (3) 100 ms after the movement onset. The same calculation was done for EvrDirCoh in the other direction. In the figure, the higher value means that more time-frequency components revealed the significant EvrDirCoh.

### *2.7.2. Pattern of change in EvrDirCoh over time*

To capture the change of EvrDirCoh over time with respect to the onset of target figure and task movement, the significant EvrDirCoh values within each time window across all the frequency bins, were summed up respectively, and plotted over time. The reason for summing up the values rather than obtaining mean was to accentuate visually the overall change of EvrDirCoh pattern that appeared on the time-frequency plane

### *2.7.3. Frequency band showing marked EvrDirCoh*

To capture what frequency band revealed marked EvrDirCoh, the rate of significant EvrDirCoh was calculated by the number of time-frequency components, within the frequency band, showing the significant EvrDirCoh, divided by the total number of time-frequency components within the corresponding frequency band. The rate was obtained for each of the focused electrode by all the time-frequency plots across all the electrode combinations.

## 3. Results

### 3.1. The maximum aperture

The perception about the size of the target figure was examined in terms of the maximum angle of the index finger metacarpophalangeal joint during the aperture motion. A 2×2 repeated-measure ANOVA with the main effects of the tasks (*Grasping* and *Matching*) and the objects (*Neutral* figure and *Ebbinghaus* figure) revealed the significant main effects of the task ($F(1, 9) = 5.098$, $p = .050$) and the target figure ($F(1, 9) = 6.089$, $p = .036$) with no interaction effect between them ($F(1, 9) = 0.112$, $p = .75$). The maximum aperture angle was smaller for the *Ebbinghaus* figure than for the *Neutral* figure and smaller in *Grasping* than in *Matching* (Figure 4).

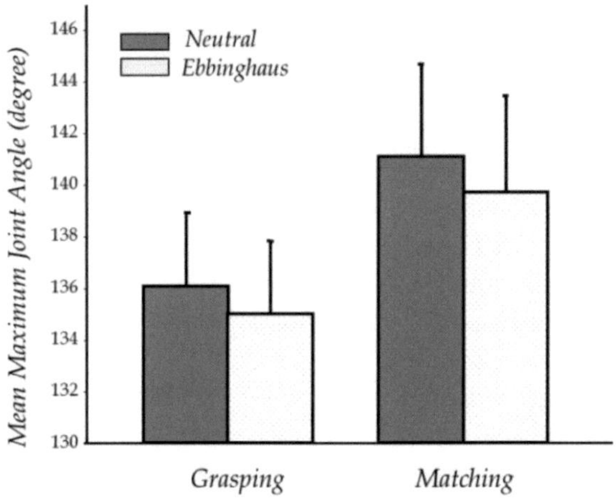


**Figure 4.** Maximum angle of the metacarpophalangeal joint as a measure of the maximum aperture during the task execution. An error bar refers to the standard error of the mean.

## 3.2. ERS/ERD with respect to the target onset

Figure 5-a shows exemplary spectrograms in F3, FC3, C3, CP3, P3, PO3, and O1 with respect to the target onset in *Grasping* performed to *Neutral* figure. According to the change in ERSP over time in the figures, increase of power spectra (ERS) within a lower frequency band (delta- and theta-bands) appeared immediately after the target onset. The decrease of the spectra (ERD) around the alpha-band frequency was also observed. This ERS-ERD pattern was mainly distributed in the parietal and occipital regions (O1, PO3, and P3 in Figure 5-a), than in frontal regions (F3 , FC3 and C3 in Figure 5-a). These ERS and ERD were significantly different from the baseline spectra. According to the analysis conducted in the previous study by the author and his colleagues (Katsumata et al., 2009: Table 1), the timing of these ERSP with respect to the target onset was 74±32 ms in the delta-ERS and 81±26 ms in the theta-RES, which were followed by the alpha- and beta-ERD (215±59 ms and 148±30 ms, respectively).

## 3.3. *ERS/ERD* with respect to the movement onset

Exemplary spectrograms with respect to the movement onset in *Grasping* and *Matching* to the *Neutral* figure were shown in Figure 5-b and 5-c respectively. Before the movement onset, the lower frequency ERS were observed in the frontal and central regions. Prominent ERD at around the alpha-band was observed in the central and parietal regions before and during the movement in both of *Grasping* and *Matching*. The prominent feature in *Grasping* was the gamma-band ERS, which appeared before the movement onset in the parietal and occipital regions and continued during the movement execution. As opposed to it, in *Matching*, the higher frequency power spectra did not reveal any change during the movement. According to the previous study (Katsumata et al., 2009: Table 1), the ERD started to increase, on average, 129±88ms in the central-parietal regions and 78±52ms in the frontal region before the movement onset and the ERS occurred 214±9 ms before the movement onset. The comparison of ERSP between *Grasping* and *Matching* revealed the significant difference in the parietal-occipital regions at the gamma-band (Figure 5-d).

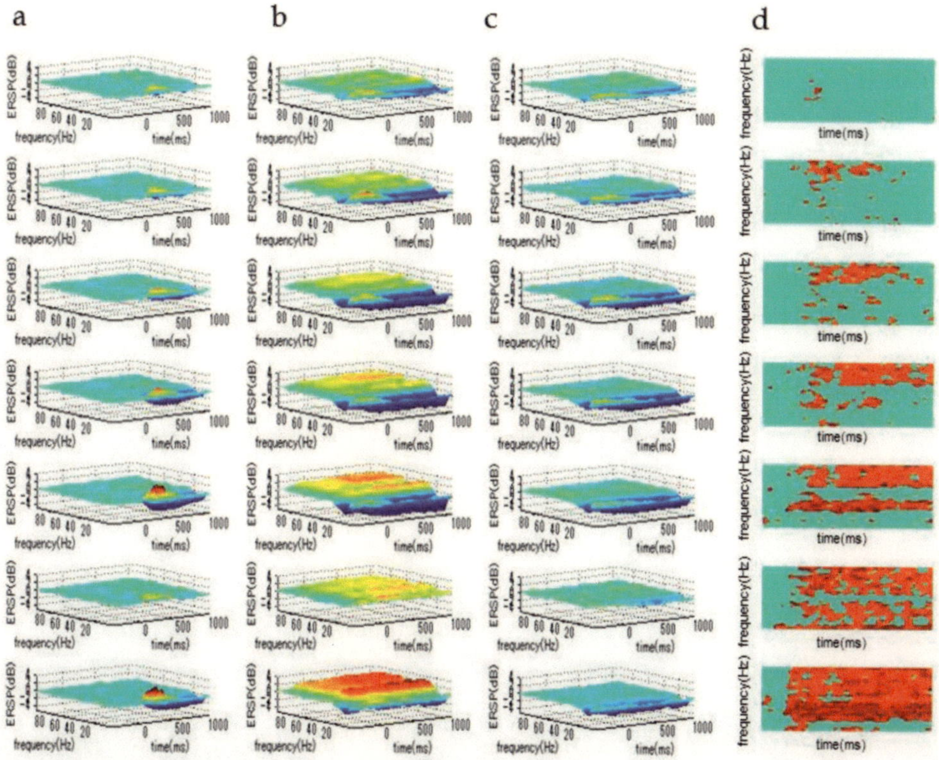


**Figure 5.** ERSP spectrograms
*Grasping* to *Neutral* figure with respect to the target onset (a), the movement onset (b), *Matching* to Neutral figure with respect to the movement onset (c), and the statistical test of the *Grasping-Matching* ERSP comparison (d). In (d), x and y axis correspond to the time and frequency of the spectrograms, respectively. The time-frequency components with the significant difference were shown in red. For each column, each plot refers to F3, FC3, C3, CP3, P3, PO3, P3, and O1, from the top to the bottom.

In summary, both of *Grasping* and *Matching* performances were affected by the illusory object, according to the aperture joint angle. In execution of the task performances, the alpha-wave ERD were observed and it did not show a notable difference between *Grasping* and *Matching*. The task-dependent difference was the gamma-wave ERS that was observed in *Grasping* but not in *Matching*.

### 3.4. Electrode combinations showing the marked coherence (EvDirCoh)

The rate of significant EvDirCoh on each time-frequency plane across electrode combinations was visualized in Figure 7 to Figure 9. Based on these figures, the results of electrode combinations that showed the characteristics of remarked coherences were reported as below. Refer to Figure 6 for the electrode locations on the left-hemisphere, which correspond to the location of each cell on the plot. Figure 7 shows the rate of significant EvDirCoh after the target onset, and Figure 8 and Figure 9 show the rate before and after the movement onset (i.e., the movement preparation and execution phase), respectively.

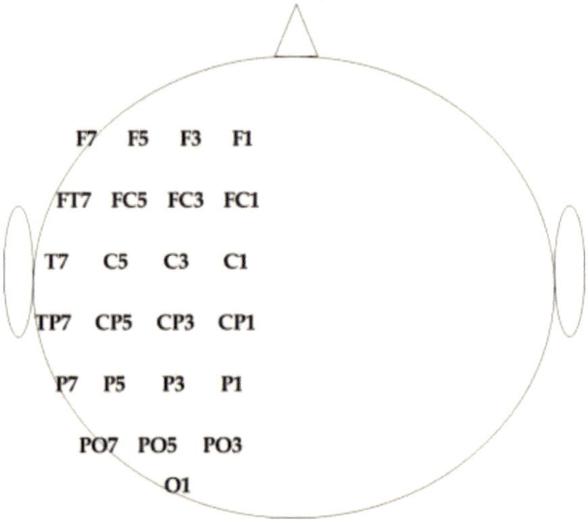


**Figure 6.** Electrode locations

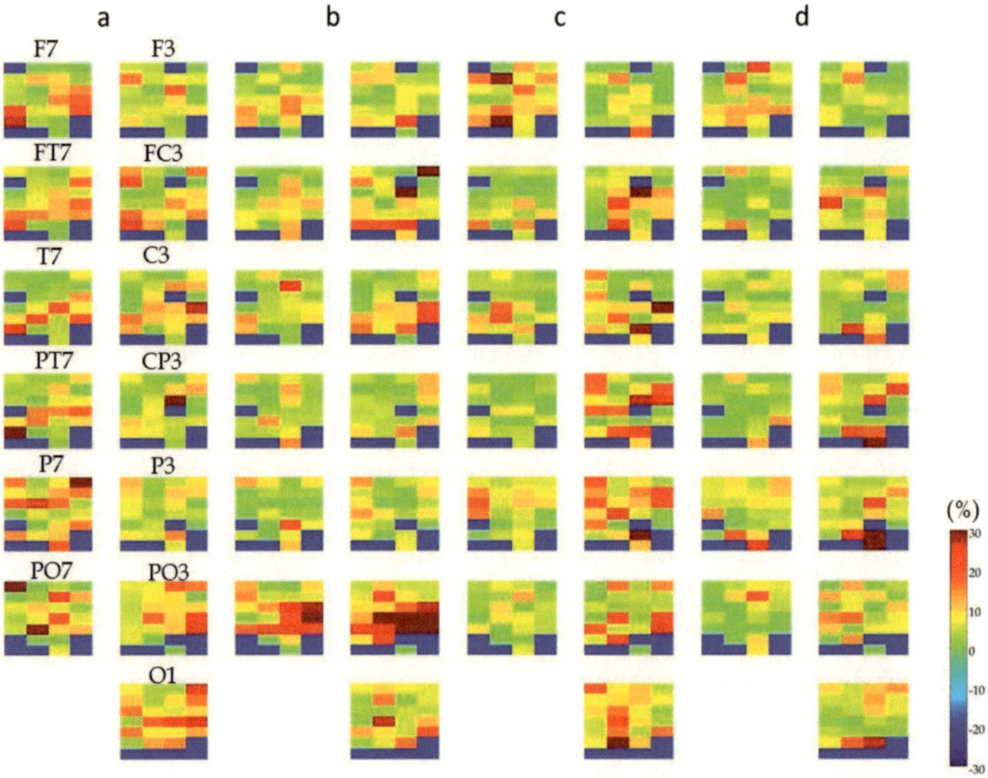


**Figure 7.** The rate of significant EvDirCoh with respect to the target onset

Coherences to other electrodes in *Grasping* (a), in *Matching* (b), from other electrodes in *Grasping* (c), *Matching* (d). Each plot shows each electrode, as shown in the left column. Higher rate of EvDirCoh was shown with red and no-significance with light green. The cells with blue refer to no electrode or the location of corresponding electrode.

### 3.4.1. *The occipital region (O1) in response to the target onset and during the movement production*

As appeared in O1, prominent EvDirCoh were observed after the onset of target figured, which implies response to the visual input about the target. The coherences between O1 and other sites were more prominent in response to the visual target, after which those were restricted to a few electrodes. In *Grasping,* the coherence from O1 to the occipito-parietal/inferior parietal region (CP1/CP3/CP5/P1/P3/ PO3/PO5/P5) was observed after the target onset and lasted for the movement execution. EvDirCoh to T7and P7 (the ventral stream) was observed, and EvDirCoh to P7 lasted for the movement execution. EvDirCoh from the inferior-parietal/superior-temporal region (PO5/P5/CP5) was observed. EvDirCoh in *Matching* appeared to be less remarkable, compared to those in *Grasping,* except for EvDirCoh to CP5 and P1/PO3 after the target onset and from PO5/PO3 after the target onset and during the movement.

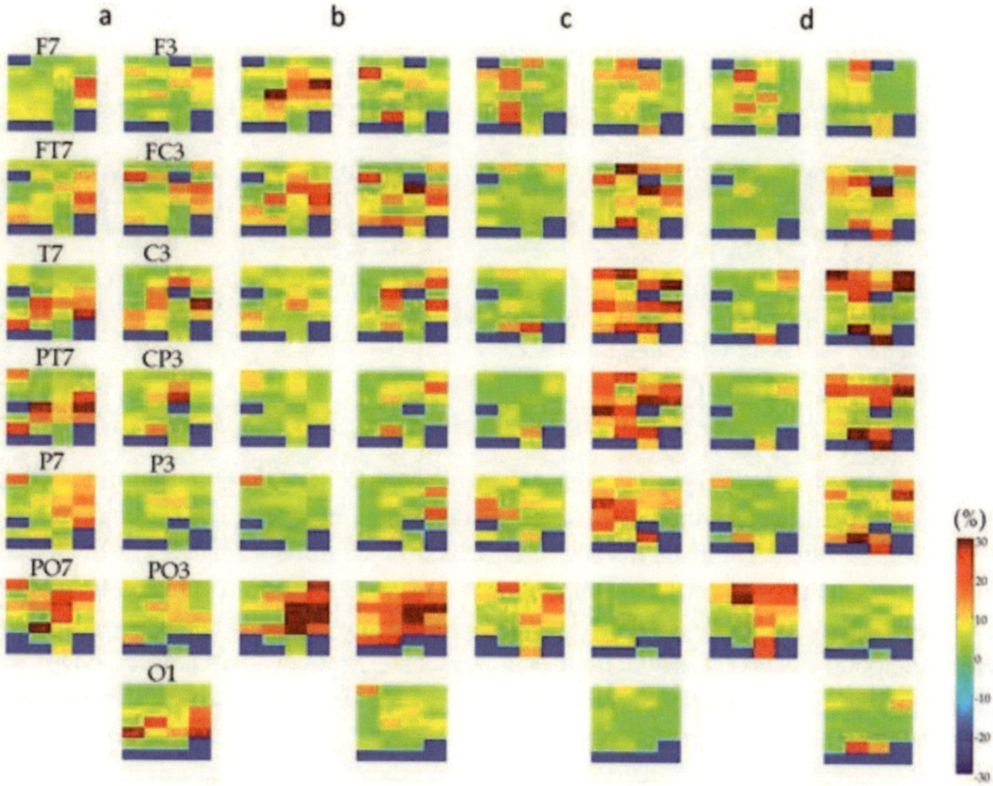


**Figure 8.** The rate of significant EvDirCoh before the movement onset
The description of the figure is the same as in Fig.7.

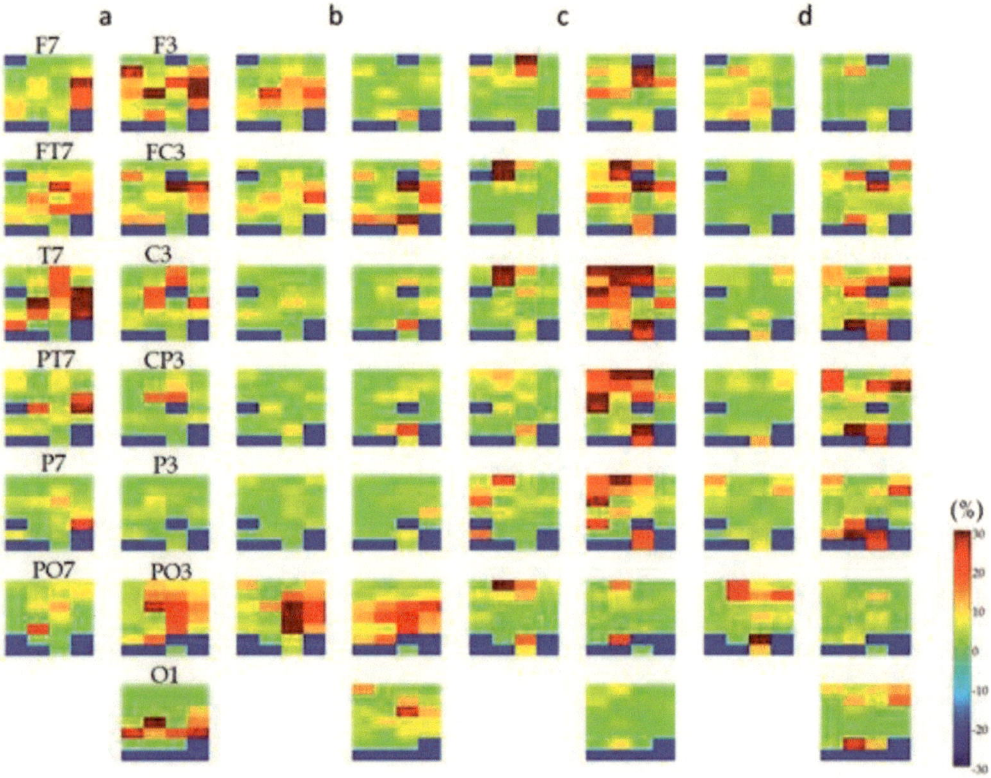


**Figure 9.** The rate of significant EvDirCoh after the movement onset
The description of the figure is the same as in Fig.7.

### *3.4.2. Electrodes relevant to the dorsal stream of visual processing (PO3, P3, and CP3)*

After the target onset, in *Grasping*, the prominent EvDirCohs were observed in P3, CP3, and PO3, which were from the divergent areas including the inferior-frontal region (F7/FT7), the medial-central region (FC1/FC3/C1/C3), the temporal region (T7/CP5), and the parieto-occipital region (PO3/PO5). Before the movement onset, EvDirCoh to PO3/P3 from the frontal, temporal, and parietal regions became more prominent, and these frontal/temporal EvDirCoh lasted for the movement execution. In *Matching*, EvDirCoh from PO3 to the parietal-occipital and posterior-temporal regions, as well as the coherence from the occipito-parietal region (O1/PO3/PO5) to P3/CP5 appeared to be remarkable. Before the movement onset, EvDirCoh from PO3 to the divergent areas, particularly the central-parietal region, became prominent, and lasted for the movement execution. EvDirCoh from the frontal region to CP3 and EvDirCoh from the parieto-occipital region to CP3/P3 were also remarkable.

#### *3.4.3. Electrodes relevant to the ventral stream of visual processing (PO7, P7, TP7, and T7)*

After the target onset, PO7/P7/PT7/T7 in *Grasping* showed EvDirCoh to electrodes in different locations and P7 and T7 received EvDirCoh from their neighborhoods, FT7/T7/PT7 or CP5/P5, respectively. Furthermore, during the movement execution, EvDirCoh from T7 to the frontal, central, and parietal regions were pronounced. EvDirCoh to T7 form the frontal region (F5/FC5) was also remarked. As for *Matching*, PO7 showed the pronounced EvDirCoh to the central and parietal regions after the target onset. Whilst these EvDirCohs became more prominent and extended to the frontal region before the movement was initiated, PO7 also showed the coherence from the frontal and the parieto-occipital region. This PO7-to-central/parietal and the frontal-to-PO7 EvDirCoh lasted during the task execution.

#### *3.4.4. Electrodes located on the frontal region (F7, F3, FC3, and FT7)*

After the target onset, EvDirCoh from F7/FT7/FC3 to posterior temporal region (PO7/P7) was observed in *Grasping*. *Matching* did not show such prominent EvDirCoh as in *Grasping*, except for EvDirCoh from FC3 to the parieto-occipital region (PO7/PO5/PO3). Before the movement was initiated, FT7 and F7 in *Matching* showed the remarked EvDirCoh to the central-parietal region, whilst the F7 in Grasping received EvDirCoh from FC5/C5 and PO5/P5. FC3 showed EvDirCoh to/from divergent areas. During the movement execution, EvDirCoh to the central-parietal region, which were centered the medial region, were observed in *Grasping*. FC3 in Grasping showed the prominent EvDirCoh from the frontal, central and temporal regions. EvDirCoh in *Matching* during the movement execution were less remarked than in *Grasping*, except for EvDirCoh from FC3 to C1/C3/CP1/PO3.

#### *3.4.5. The electrode located on the motor cortex for movement production (C3)*

The focus of coherence in C3 is on the preparation and execution of task movements. The remarkable feature before the movement initiation was that C3 received EvDirCoh from divergent areas in *Grasping*, which contrasts to EvDirCoh in *Matching* mainly from the frontal region. During the movement, EvDirCoh to C3 in *Grasping* became pronounced and centred in the frontal and temporal regions.

### 3.5. Coherence profile over time

According to Figure 10, all most all of the analyzed electrodes showed increase in the coherence after the target onset, which lasted for 500-600 ms. This indicates that there were communications across different cortical sites, possibly for processing information about the target figure for the up-coming task execution. Regardless of task conditions (*Grasping* or *Matching*), the electrodes that are associated with either of the dorsal or ventral stream showed the increase of coherence, which indicates that both of the streams might be involved in the visual processing about the target figure. The pattern of coherence over time with respect to the onset of task movement was as follows.

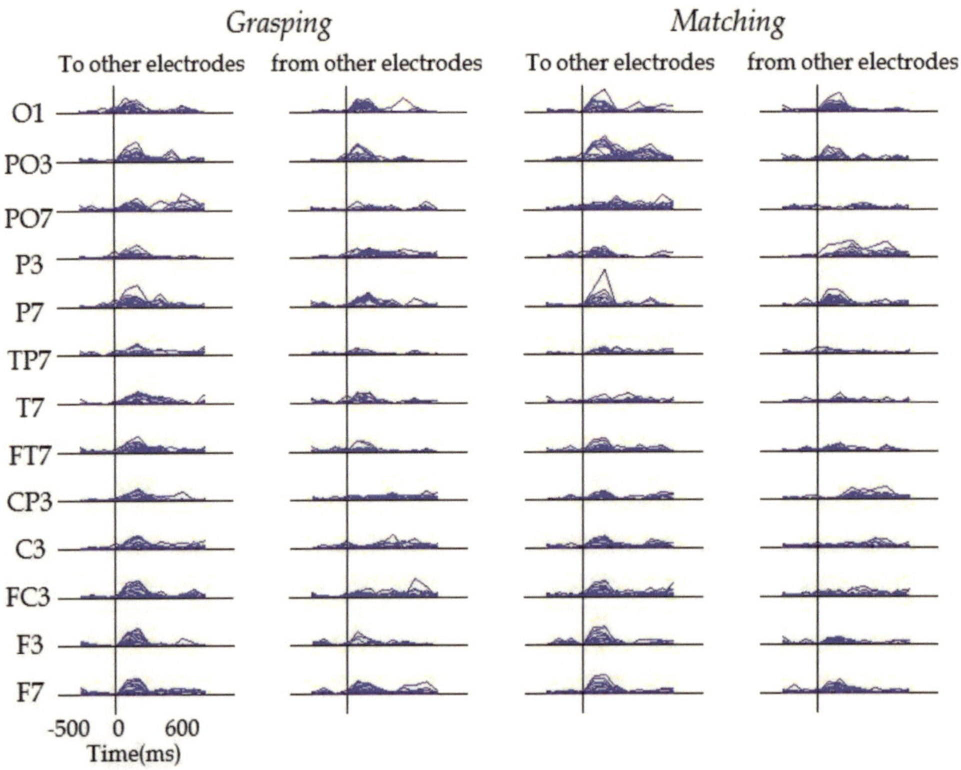


**Figure 10.** Change of EvDirCoh over time with respect to the target onset
23 EvDirCoh profiles to/from other channels were superposed in each plot. Only the positive part of EvDirCoh, which was significantly larger than the baseline, was shown. Each line indicates how the positive EvDirCoh was prominent within each time window on the time-frequency plot.

O1 that corresponds to the visual cortex in the left-hemisphere showed the increase in some of coherences before the initiation of the movement and lasted during the movement execution. This was remarked in *Grasping*, compared to those in *Matching*. Before the movement onset in *Grasping*, increase of coherence was observed in PO7, P7, FT7, CP3, FC3, and F7. This was followed by the coherence increase in TP7, P3, and T7 at the movement onset. The increase of coherence was also observed before the maximum aperture was produced (e.g., T7, CP3, C3, FC3, and F3), and after the peak aperture (e.g., PO3, PO7, P3, TP7, T7, FT7, and CP3). According to the timing of these coherences, there seem to be temporal pattern of coherence change from the preparation of movement to the movement completion. For instance, the increase of coherence in PO7 and P7 before the movement onset was followed by TP7and T7 at around the movement onset, and FT7 after the peak aperture production (the 1st column of Figure 11), which seems to reflect the activity of the ventral stream. Likewise, the increase of coherence in PO3 before the movement onset was followed by P3 at around the onset, and CP3 after the peak aperture production (the 2nd column of Figure 11), which seems to reflect the activity of the dorsal stream.

As for *Matching*, according to the appearance about Figure 11, there were less remarked increases of coherences, compared to those in *Grasping*. The remarked increase of coherence in O1 was observed after the movement onset. Before the initiation of movement, the increase of coherence was observed in PO3, PO7, T7, FT7, C3, FC3, F3, and F7. From the movement onset to the moment of the peak aperture, coherence of PO3, PO7, P3, CP3, C3, and FC3 showed remarked increase. After the peak aperture, the increase of coherence was observed in PO3, PO7, P3, TP7, T7, and CP3. These coherence patterns indicate that *Matching* movement was executed with less connections or communications among the cortical sites, compared to *Grasping*.

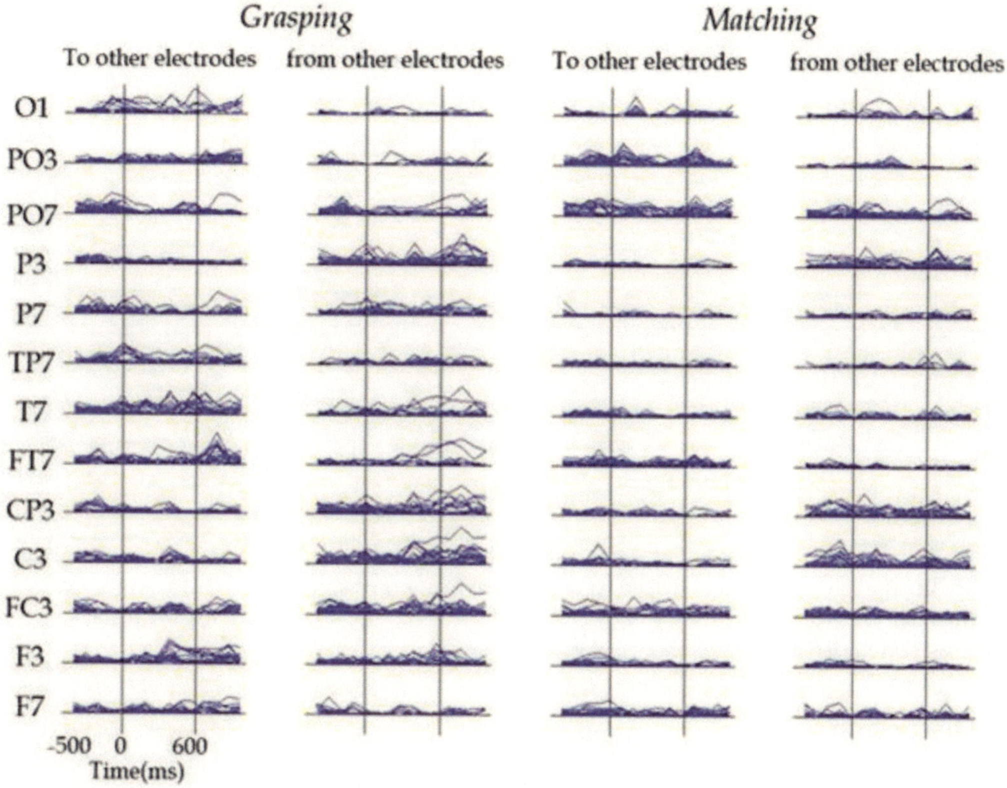


**Figure 11.** Change of EvDirCoh over time with respect to the movement onset
Description of the figure is the same as Figure 10.

## 3.6. Frequency band showing the remarked coherence

Figure 12 shows the rate of significant EvDirCoh within each frequency band. In this figure, higher value indicates that more time-frequency components revealed significant EvDirCoh within corresponding frequency band. The figure can also indicate what frequency band was dominant across all the frequency bands.

With respect to the target onset, the lower frequency bands (delta, theta, and alpha) appeared to be more dominant compared to the beta, gamma, and higher gamma bands in the most of electrodes. Some of the electrodes in *Matching* (e.g., PO3 and PO7) revealed higher rate of significant time-frequency components in higher frequency bands. As opposed to it, with respect to the movement onset, the rate of higher frequency band (gamma and/or higher gamma) increased, which was particularly prominent in CP3, C3, FC3, PO3, PO7, P3, P7, and T7 in *Grasping* and/or *Matching*.

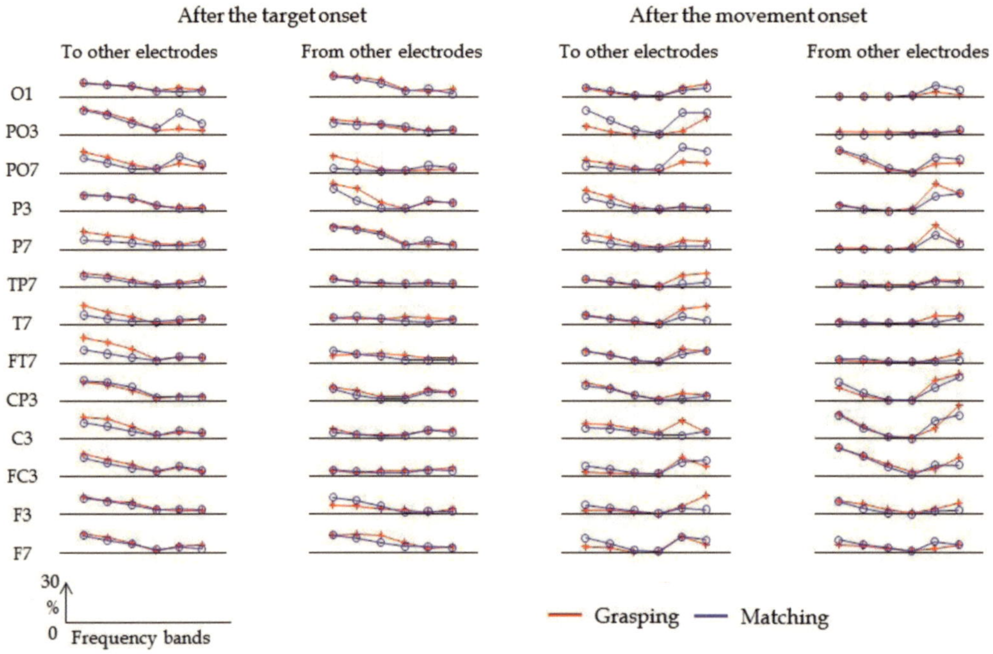


**Figure 12.** The rate of significant EvDirCoh within each frequency band
Each symbol refers to each frequency band, such as, delta, theta, alpha, beta, gamma, and higher-gamma, from the left to the right on each plot.

## 4. Discussion

### 4.1. The size-illusion effect for *Grasping* and *Matching*

The comparison of task performances in terms of the peak aperture angle showed a significant difference between the tasks (*Grasping* and *Matching*) as well as between the task-objects (*Neutral* and *Ebbinghaus figure*). This indicated that not only *Matching* but also *Grasping* was affected by the size illusion. This implies that the cognitive processing about the size perception was also involved in the performances in *Grasping*. The *Grasping-Matching* difference in the illusion effect can imply the different magnitude of the illusion effect and/or the task-dependent difference in scaling relationship between the perceived object size and the produced aperture size. In other words, the cognitive processing for shaping the aperture based on the size perception may not be exactly the same in these two task executions.

The effect of visual illusion on a prehensile movement task to the illusory object as well as on a perceptual discrimination task have also reported in some earlier studies (e.g., Franz et al., 2000, 2001; Glover & Dixon, 2002; Mendoza et al., 2005), which contradicts to the hypothesis of dissociative systems for perception and action by the ventral/ dorsal stream (Aglioti et al., 1995; Goodale & Jakobson, 1992; Haffenden & Goodale, 1998). These illusion effects are attributed to the task conditions, such as, complex target figures (McIntosh et al., 2004), movement production in an open-loop manner (i.e., movements to a remembered object: Heath et al., 2005; Westwood et al., 2000a), and online reorganization of the grasping aperture in response to the change of object size (Heath et al., 2006b). These findings have led to arguments such that: the motor system integrates the ventral and dorsal streams (Ellis et al., 1999); the sensorimotor system can operate independently of the cognitive/perceptual system (Flanagan & Beltzner, 2000); a prehensile movement is produced through multiple visuomotor processes (Westwood et al., 2000b); the ventral stream has connection to the prefrontal areas and, thereby, it may associate with the visuomotor control of a prehensile action (Lee & van Donkelaar, 2002); and online prehensile control may be produced through egocentric and allocentric visual information processing (Heath et al., 2006a).

Even though there are functionally and anatomically distinctive visual pathways at the cortical level, executing a visuomotor task may be achieved through an integrative process of these pathways. These visual pathways may be involved differentially in task-dependent manner. For instance, if a pure visual discrimination task such that participants are asked to discern which of two objects looks larger/smaller, it is expected that a cortical activity associated with the ventral stream may be dominant (Farrer et al., 2002; Westwod et al., 2000b). Likewise, if reaching or grasping needs to be produced in an open-loop manner (e.g., a visual object is occluded before or right after the onset of a prehensile movement), the movement production needs to be based on the memory of the object shape (Heath et al., 2005; Westwood et al., 2000a; Westwood et al., 2000b). In these cases, the nature of task performance requires cognitive processing, which will be achieved via the ventral stream dominantly. Given the above results about the Ebbinghaus effect, cortical activation patterns revealed in ERSP and EvDirCoh need to be interpreted in terms of how cortical sites associated with the dorsal/ventral stream in an integrated fashion. In this sense, the difference in the ERSP and/or EvDirCoh pattern between *Grasping* and *Matching* may reflect the qualitative difference in the integrated cortical process with which cognitive processing is associated.

## 4.2. Comparison of ERSP pattern between the task conditions

### *4.2.1. ERD observed in Grasping and Matching*

ERD has been regarded as representing an activated cortical state and thereby sensory, motor, and/or cognitive processing is enhanced. Therefore, the cortical regions showing ERD during the task performances can be regarded as functionally associating with the perceptual-motor process for the tasks. The comparison of the ERSP patterns between *Grasping* and *Matching* revealed that the ERD pattern appeared to be virtually identical. It indicates that the cortical excitability assessed by ERD during the two perceptual-motor tasks was not distinctive. This lack of distinction in ERD between *Grasping* and *Matching* with the size-illusion effect in both the task performances suggests that the perceptual-motor process in *Grasping*, somehow, involved cognitive processing about the target figure as in *Matching*.

The ERD after the target onset were observed not only in the occipital region (i.e., visual area), but also in the central-parietal regions. This implies some visual processing rather than just responding to the visual stimulus, which could possibly be associated with the task execution. The ERD in occipital-parietal regions was observed with respect to the aperture movement onset as well as after the target onset. Based on that the posterior parietal cortex functions for the integration of the sensory information as well as the visuomotor coordination (Buneo & Andersen, 2006; Burnod et al., 1999; Culham et al., 2006; Darling et al., 2007; Stein, 1995), the occipital-parietal ERD can be interpreted that the visual information was further processed via the higher level of visual areas toward the movement execution.

The ERD in F3, F4, FC3, FC4, C3 and C4 in Figure 5 indicates that the frontal and pre-frontal areas were involved in the task execution. This frontal area ERD was observed not only in *Matching* but also *Grasping*, which indicates that the frontal cortical network may be involved in the execution of both tasks. The functional connection between the frontal area and the parietal cortex plays a role for the spatial organization of arm and hand motions, such as, reaching and grasping (Caminiti et al., 1998; Rizzolatti et al., 1997). The premotor and motor cortices function for preparing and controlling movements to achieve a given motor task goal (Kandel et al., 2000; Zigmond et al., 1999). The frontal ERD seem to indicate these functional activities for the task execution.

### *4.2.2. ERS as the characteristic of Grasping*

The notable feature in the ERSP spectrogram was the ERS observed not in *Matching* but in *Grasping*. The ERS within the higher frequency band, corresponding to the gamma-wave, started before the onset of the aperture joint motion and continued during the *Grasping* execution. The ERS was observed mainly in the occipital-parietal regions (e.g., O1, O2, OP3, OP4, P3, P4 and CP3 in Figure 5), those of which associate with sensory information processing and motor production. Originally, ERS has been regarded as the cortical state of decreased excitability and suppressed processing of specific information in underlying neuronal networks (Neuper & Pfurtscheller, 2001; Pfurtscheller, 1992). However, ERS has been observed in association with ERD and the accumulation of findings about ERS by recent studies, as described below, suggests that not only ERD but also ERS plays a role in the cortical network's function for the execution of task performances. The cortical activity pattern of ERS in association with ERD was observed, such as: The locally specific alpha- and/or beta-ERD accompanied by ERS in neighboring areas (the focal ERD/surround ERS: Gerloff et al., 1998; Neuper & Pfurtscheller, 2001; Pfurtscheller & Neuper, 1994); The mu-rhythm ERD in the motor cortex with respect to the movement onset followed by the beta-wave ERS with respect to the movement offset (Pfurtscheller et al., 1999b); and a stronger mu-rhythm ERD over the motor cortex accompanied by a smaller beta-wave ERS during manipulation of a cube (Neuper et al., 2006). Amongst those findings, the inhibitory mechanism of ERS, which is for limiting or controlling excitatory process associated with task execution, has been proposed, such as, the antagonistic ERS-ERD as a mechanism to enhance focal activation by simultaneous inhibition of the other cortical areas (Neuper & Pfurtscheller, 2001; Suffczynski et al., 1999) and the post-movement ERS as reflecting some selective attention or an active inhibition to accentuate a task-related information processing by inhibiting the task irrelevant other cortical areas (Neuper & Pfurtscheller, 2001). When a learned movement pattern was intentionally prevented from being retrieved, increase in the alpha-band task-related power (i.e., alpha-wave ERS) was observed in the primary motor cortex that indicating the inhibition (Hummel & Gerloff, 2002). ERS observed in memory process was interpreted as an inhibitory role to block a memory search from entering irrelevant parts of neural networks (Klimesch, 1996).

Given the above findings, the gamma band ERS pattern during *Grasping* can be regarded as representing the aspect of a perceptual-motor process, which is characteristic to *Grasping*. Whilst the alpha and lower beta ERS represent reduced information processing or deactivation in underlying cortical networks, the gamma band ERS has been reported during sensory encoding (Galambos et al., 1981), cognitive processing (Basar & Bullock, 1992), and movement execution (DeFrance & Sheer, 1988). These gamma band oscillations were thought to be related to binding of sensory information and integrating sensorimotor process, since binding signals at a higher level of processing may require signal transmission higher than the alpha and lower beta oscillation (Singer, 1993; Pfurtscheller, 1998). In this sense, the gamma band ERS may represent a functional mechanism beyond being inhibitory.

In this analysis, the two oscillatory components, one showing ERD and the other ERS, were observed in a single electrode in the parietal-occipital regions. Different frequency oscillations embedded at a single electrode are interpreted as one neural network generating different types of oscillations (Pfurtscheller & Lopes da Silva, 1999). Therefore, the ERD in both of *Grasping* and *Matching* and the ERS observed only in *Grasping* seem to be associated with different functional roles respectively. Considering about the nature of task execution in *Grasping* and *Matching*, the ERD pattern may represent the functional aspect common to the both of *Grasping* and *Matching* (i.e., associating the index-thumb joint motions with respect to the perception about the size of visual target), and the ERS pattern may represent the functional aspect exclusive to a visually-guided aperture organization process in *Grasping* (e.g., continuously updating the target object-hand spatial relationship to reach out and shaping the aperture).

### 4.3. Cortical communication in terms of EvDirCoh and the nature of task execution process

According to the feature of the rate of significant EvDirCoh, which captures the pattern of coherence appeared on the time-frequency plane, the following characteristic EvDirCoh was observed in each of the task performances. The coherence analysis has been applied to time series of neural system based on the assumption that the coherence reflects the functional connectivity, neural communication and/or signal transmission between two or more neural activities (Sameshima & Baccalá, 1999). The results in the present study are interpreted from this perspective.

After the target onset, the significant coherences were dominant amongst the lower frequency (the delta, theta, and alpha bands in Figure 12). This implies that the visual processing in response to the target object was achieved by the neural communication with those frequency bands. As opposed to it, the gamma and higher gamma bands became prominent after the movement onset. Those prominent frequency bands were observed particularly in CP3, C3, FC3, PO7, P3, P7, and T7 in *Grasping* and *Matching*. Since these sites are associated with the coordinate transformation and the hand movement organization, the result implies that the communication between different cortical sites occur at higher neural oscillation during the preparation and execution of task movement.

As for the temporal characteristics of EvDirCoh, the most of the analyzed electrodes showed increase in EvDirCoh after the target onset and lasted for approximately 500 ms. This EvDirCoh increase may reflect the communications across different cortical sites for processing information about the target figure for the up-coming task execution. With respect to the movement execution in *Grasping*, the increase of significant EvDirCoh was observed with the temporal order of: (1) PO3, PO7, P7, FT7, CP3, and FC3 before the movement onset; (2) P3, TP7, and T7 at round the moment of the movement onset; (3) T7, CP3, C3, FC3, and F3 during the movement execution; and (4) PO3, PO7, P3, P7, T7, FT7, CP3, C3, and FC3 after the peak aperture produced. After the movement onset and before the peak aperture production, the dorsal stream-relevant electrodes (P3 and CP3), the ventral stream-relevant electrodes (PO7, P7, T7, and FT7), the frontal region (FC3 and F3), and the motor cortex (C3) showed the increase of the coherence. This may reflect the movement execution by the cortical communication for exchanging information. These temporal patterns were less pronounced in *Matching*, even though there were increases of EvDirCoh amongst the electrodes. In both *Grasping* and *Matching*, the involvement of the dorsal/ventral stream and the frontal cortex in the preparatory and execution phases was shown in the temporally ordered fashion.

### *4.3.1. Coherence relevant to the task events (the target onset and the movement preparation-execution)*

After the target onset, the visual cortex (O1) and other areas showed coherence to/from different cortical site. This may implies the response to the visual target. Particularly, the parietal-occipital region (PO3 and PO7) in *Matching* showed the prominent coherence to the parietal, occipital, and posterior temporal regions. This means that there were functional connections within these regions, which can be possibly associated with the visual information transmission from the visual cortex to the higher level of visual processing. Since executing the *Matching* task requires estimating the center circle size, which was potentially achieved by combining the information about the surrounding circles, information processing in *Matching* can be more demanding than in *Grasping*.

In the movement preparation phase, PO7 and PO3 in *Matching* showed the prominent coherences as in the target onset phase. Furthermore, PO7 and CP3 showed the connection from the frontal region, whilst the frontal region showed connection to different sites. These characteristics may reflect the cortical communication for visual processing and movement preparation. As for *Grasping*, the prominent characteristics were the connection to the central and parietal regions (C3, CP3 and P3) from divergent areas, mainly the inferior frontal, frontal, and temporal regions. Since the parietal region plays a functional role for coordinate transfer to organize a limb movement, these coherence pattern may reflect this functional activity. Another feature was the connection from electrode associated with the ventral stream, PO7, PT7, and T7 to the central-parietal region. As described above, different EvDirCoh patterns were observed in the preparatory phase before initiating the task movement.

The remarkable feature of EvDirCoh in *Grasping* for executing the movement was observed in the connection to frontal-central region (FC3/C3/CP3) from inferior frontal, frontal, and temporal regions. Furthermore, the connection from the temporal (T7) and frontal (FT7/F7/F3/FC3) to the central and frontal region became more prominent than in the preparatory phase. As opposed to it, in *Matching*, the remarked coherence was observed in restricted sites, which were similar to that in the preparatory phase. This indicates that executing the task movement was achieved through more active cortical communications in *Grasping*, compared to in *Matching*. The movement of reaching and grasping requires the perceptual-motor process to organize a limb movement, whilst the size-mating task is executed only by producing the index finger-thumb motion. Such difference can be reflected in the P3/CP3/C3 characteristics in *Grasping*. Contrary to it, the process of assessing the object size and associating the perceived size with a particular finger motion is a central part of *Matching*, and this aspect might be reflected in the target onset and preparatory phases.

### 4.3.2. *EvDirCoh characteristics associated with the dorsal/ventral streams*

The visual information from the primary visual cortex is transmitted further via the dorsal stream to the middle temporal area and the medial superior temporal area, as well as via the ventral stream to the posterior inferior temporal cortex and the anterior inferior temporal cortex (Kandel et al., 2000; Zigmond et al., 1999). The electrodes PO3, P3, and CP3 are relevant to the dorsal stream, and PO7, P7, TP7, and T7 to the ventral stream. In the present study, EvDirCoh patterns associated with these electrodes showed following characteristics. In *Grasping*, PO7, P7, TP7, and particularly T7 (the ventral stream) showed the marked connection mainly to the frontal and central regions during the task execution. P3 and CP3 (the dorsal stream) also showed the connection from the frontal and temporal regions, especially in the preparatory and execution phases. Since the *Grasping* performance was also affected by the size-illusion, this result does not contradict to the idea of the cognitive role of the ventral stream. As opposed to it, in *Matching*, T7 and FT7 did not show the remarked coherence, even though PO3 and PO7 revealed the marked coherence during the task execution.

These results revealed that the involvement of the dorsal and ventral streams for the task execution was not exclusive between *Matching* and *Grasping*. But the patterns of EvDirCoh were different between them, which suggest that the involvement of the cortical stream and the cortical communication are task-dependent. The analysis of ERSP did not reveal the detail of cortical activation pattern as shown by EvDirCoh, even though it could demonstrate the task dependent characteristics of cortical activity. Difference between these analyses is that ERSP, as well as other analytical measure (e.g., hemodynamics in fMRI and the event-related potential in EEG) examine the amount or magnitude of neuronal actvity, whilst coherence takes care of the relationship between two or more neural activities. Therefore, information about the cortical activities, which is more than the amount, can be available. This aspect seems to be attributed to the findings reported above. The present study could reveal the characteristics of cortical activity and communication, which could be dependent on the nature of the perceptual-motor process in the task execution. Further studies are necessary for investigating what task situations/conditions can induce the ERSP/EvDirCoh characteristics and how those are associated with the involvement of cognitive processing for a perceptual-motor task.

## 5. Conclusion

The involvement of cognitive processing in the perceptual-motor process for achieving a motor task goal was examined by *Grasping* and *Matching* tasks, in terms of cortical activity. To this end, the event-related spectral perturbation and directed coherence were analyzed. Those analyses could reveal the different cortical activation and communication pattern, which could be attributed to the difference in the nature of perceptual-motor process in these tasks.

## Author details

Hiromu Katsumata
*Daito Bunka University, Japan*

## Acknowledgement

This study was founded by the Grant-in-Aid for Scientific Research (#20500507) in Japan Society for the Promotion of Science, and the Research Grant in Daito-Bunka University (#220102). EEG data collection was conducted by the support of Dr. Kuniyasu Imanaka and his doctoral students at Tokyo Metropolitan University.

## 6. References

Aglioti, S., DeSouza, J.F.X.& Goodale, M.A. (1995). Size-contrast illusions deceive the eye but not the hand. *Current Biology*, Vol.5, pp. 679-685,

Basar, E.& Bullock, T.H. (1992). *Induced Rhythms in the Brain*. Birkhäuser, Basel

Buneo, C.A.& Andersen, R.A. (2006). The posterior parietal cortex: Sensorimotor interface for the planning and online control of visually guided movements. *Neuropsychologia*, Vol.44, pp. 2594-2606,

Burnod, Y., Baraduc, P., Battaglia-Mayer, A., Guigon, E., Koechlin, E., Ferraina, S., Lacquaniti, F.& Caminiti, R. (1999). Parieto-frontal coding of reaching: An integrated framework. *Experimental Brain Research*, Vol.129, pp. 325-346,

Caminiti, R., Ferraina, S.& Mayer, A.B. (1998). Visuomotor transformations: early cortical mechanisms of reaching. *Current Opinion in Neurobiology*, Vol.8, pp. 753-761,

Culham, J.C., Cavina-Pratesi, C.& Singhal, A. (2006). The role of parietal cortex in visuomotor control: What have we learned from neuroimaging? *Neuropsychologia*, Vol.44, pp. 2668-2684,

Darling, W.G., Seitz, R.J., Peltier, S.S., Tellmann, L.& Butler, A. (2007). Visual cortex activation in kinesthetic guidance of reaching. *Experimental Brain Research*, Vol.179, No.4, pp. 607-619,

DeFrance, J.& Sheer, D.E. (1988). Focused arousal, 40-Hz EEG and motor programming. In: *The EEG of Mental Activities*, D. Giannitrapani & K. Murri (Eds), 153-168, Karger, Basel

Delorme, A.& Makeig, S. (2004). EEGLAB: an open source toolbox for analysis of single-trial EEG dynamics including independent component analysis. *Journal of Neuroscience Methods*, Vol.134, pp. 9-21,

Ellis, R.R., Flanagan, J.R.& Lederman, S.J. (1999). The influence of visual illusions on grasp position. *Experimental Brain Research*, Vol.125, pp. 109-114,

Flanagan, J.R.& Beltzner, M.A. (2000). Independence of perceptual and sensorimotor predictions in the size-weight illusion. *Nature Neuroscience*, Vol.3, No.7, pp. 737-741,

Franz, V.H., Fahle, M., Bulthoff, H.H.& Gegenfurtner, K.R. (2001). Effects of visual illusions on grasping. *Journal of Experimental Psychology: Human Perception and Performance*, Vol.27, No.5, pp. 1124-1144,

Franz, V.H., Gegenfurtner, K.R., Bulthoff, H.H.& Fahle, M. (2000). Grasping visual illusions: No evidence for a dissociation between perception and action. *Psychological Science*, Vol.11, No.1, pp. 20-25,

Galambos, R., Makeig, S.& Talmachoff, P.J. (1981). A 40-Hz auditory potential recorded from the human scalp. *Proceedings of the National Academy of Sciences*, Vol.78, pp. 2643-2647,

Gerloff, C., Hadley, J., Richard, J., Uenishi, N., Honda, M.& Hallett, M. (1998). Functional coupling and regional activation of human cortical motor areas during simple, internally paced and externally paced finger movements. *Brain*, Vol.121, pp. 1513-1531,

Glover, S.& Dixon, P. (2002). Dynamic effects of the Ebbinghaus illusion in grasping: Support for a planning/control model of action. *Perception and Psychophysics*, Vol.64, No.2, pp. 266-278,

Goodale, M.A., & Jakobson, L.S. (1992). Action systems in the posterior parietal cortex. *Behavioral and Brain Sciences*, Vol.15, No.4, pp. 747,

Goodale, M.A., & Milner, A.D. (1992). Separate visual pathways for perception and action. *Trends in Neuroscience*, Vol.15, No.1, pp. 20-25,

Goodale, M.A., Meenan, J.P., Bulthoff, H.H., Nicolle, D.A., Murphy, K.J.& Racicot, C.I. (1994). Separate neural pathways for the visual analysis of object shape in perception and prehension. *Current Biology*, Vol.4, No.7, pp. 604-610,

Haffenden, A.M.& Goodale, M.A. (1998). The effect of pictorial illusion on prehension and perception. *Journal of Cognitive Neuroscience*, Vol.10, No.1, pp. 122-136,

Haggard, P.& Wing, A. (1995). Coordinated responses following mechanical perturbation of the arm during prehension. *Experimental Brain Research*, Vol.102, pp. 483-494,

Heath, M., Rival, C.& Neely, K. (2006a). Visual feedback schedules influence visuomotor resistance to the Muller-Lyer figures. *Experimental Brain Research*, Vol.168, No.3, pp. 348-356,

Heath, M., Rival, C., Neely, K.& Krigolson, O. (2006b). Muller-Lyer figures influence the online reorganization of visually guided grasping movements. *Experimental Brain Research*, Vol.169, No.4, pp. 473-481,

Heath, M., Westwood, D.A., Rival, C.& Neely, K. (2005). Time course analysis of closed- and open-loop grasping of the Muller-Lyer illusion. *Journal of Motor Behavior*, Vol.37, No.3, pp. 179-185,

Hummel, F.C., Andres, F., Altenmuller, E., Dichgans, J.& Gerloff, C. (2002). Inhibitory control of acquired motor programs in the human brain. *Brain*, Vol.125, pp. 404-420,

Jeannerod, M. (1981). Intersegmental coordination during reaching at natural visual objects. In: *Attention and performance*, J. Long & A. Baddeley (Eds), Vol. 9, pp. 153-168, Erlbaum, Hillsdale, NJ

Jeannerod, M. (1984). The timing of natural prehension movements. *Journal of Motor Behavior*, Vol.16, pp. 235-254,

Kamitake, T., Harashima, H., Miyakawa, H., & Saito, Y. (1984). A time-series analysis method based on the directed transinformation. *Electron. Commun. Jap.*, Vol.67, pp. 1-9,

Kandel, E.R., Schwartz, J.H.& Jessell, T.M. (2000). *Principles of Neural Science*. McGraw-Hill, New York

Katsumata, H., Suzuki, K., Tanaka, T. & Imanaka, K. (2009). The involvement of cognitive processing in a perceptual-motor process examined with EEG time-frequency analysis. *Clinical Neurophysiology*, Vol.120, pp. 484-496,

Kelso, J.A.S. (1995). *Dynamic Patterns: the self-organization of brain and behavior*. The MIT press, Cambridge, Massachusetts

Klimesch, W. (1996). Memory processes, brain oscillations and EEG synchronization. *Journal of Psychophysiology*, Vol.24, pp. 61-100,

Lee, D.N. (1980). Visuo-motor coordination in space-time. In: *Tutorials in Motor Behavior*, G.E. Stelmach & J. Requin (Eds), 281-295, North-Holland Pub., Amsterdam

Lee, J.-H.& van Donkelaar, P. (2002). Dorsal and ventral visual stream contributions to perception-action interactions during pointing. *Experimental Brain Research*, Vol.143, pp. 440-446,

Makeig, S. (1993). Auditory event-related dynamics of the EEG spectrum and effects of exposure to tones. *Electroencephalography and clinical Neurophysiology*, Vol.86, pp. 283-293,

McIntosh, R.D., Dijkerman, H.C., Mon-Williams, M.& Milner, A.D. (2004). Grasping what is graspable: Evidence from visual form agnosia. *Cortex*, Vol.40, pp. 695-702,

Mendoza, J., Hansen, S., Glazebrook, C.M., Keetch, K.M.& Elliott, D. (2005). Visual illusions affect both movement planning and on-line control: A multiple cue position on bias and goal-directed action. *Human Movement Science*, Vol.24, pp. 760-773,

Neuper, C.& Pfurtscheller, G. (2001). Event-related dynamics of cortical rhythms: Frequency-specific features and functional correlates. *International Journal of Psychophysiology*, Vol.43, pp. 41-58,

Neuper, C., Wortz, M.& Pfurtscheller, G. (2006). ERD/ERS patterns reflecting sensorimotor activation and deactivation. In: *Progress in Brain Research*, C. Neuper & W. Klimesch (Eds), Vol. 159, pp. 211-222, Elsevier

Pfurtscheller, G. (1992). Event-related synchronization (ERS): an electrophysiological correlate of cortical areas at rest. *Electroencephalography and Clinical Neurophysiology*, Vol.82, pp. 62-69,

Pfurtscheller, G. (1998). EEG event-related desynchronization (ERD) and event-related synchronization (ERS). In: *Electroencephalography: Basic Principles, Clinical Applications and Related Fields, 4th Edition.*, E. Niedermeyer & F.H. Lopes da Silva (Eds). 958-967, Williams and Wilkins, Baltimore, MD

Pfurtscheller, G. (2001). Functional brain imaging based on ERD/ERS. *Vision Research*, Vol.41, pp. 1257-1260,

Pfurtscheller, G.& Andrew, C. (1999). Event-related changes of band power and coherence: Methodology and interpretation. *Journal of Clinical Neurophysiology*, Vol.16, No.6, pp. 512,

Pfurtscheller, G.& Lopes da Silva, F.H. (1999a). *Event-Related Desynchronization*. Elsevier Science, Amsterdam

Pfurtscheller, G.& Lopes da Silva, F.H. (1999b). Functional meaning of event-related desynchronization (ERD) and synchronization (ERS). In: *Event-Related Desynchronization: Handbook of Electroencephalography and Clinical Neurophysiology*, G. Pfurtscheller & F.H. Lopes da Silva (Eds), Vol .6, pp. 51-65, Elsevier Science, Amsterdam

Pfurtscheller, G.& Neuper, C. (1994). Event-related synchronization of mu rhythm in the EEG over the cortical hand area in man. *Neuroscience Letter*, Vol.174, pp. 93-96,

Ranganathan, R.& Carlton, L.G. (2007). Perception-action coupling and anticipatory performance in baseball batting. *Journal of Motor Behavior*, Vol.39, No.5, pp. 369-380,

Rizzolatti, G., Fogassi, L.& Gallese, V. (1997). Parietal cortex: from sight to action. *Current Opinion in Neurobiology*, Vol.7, No.4, pp. 562-567,

Saito, Y. & Harashima, H. (1981). Tracking of information within multichannel EEG record-causal analysis in EEG. In: *Recent Advances in EEG and Meg data processing*, Yamaguchi, N. & Fujisawa, K. (Eds), 133-146, Elsevier, Amsterdam

Sameshima, K.& Baccalá, L.A. (1999). Using partial directed coherence to describe neuronal ensemble interactions. *Journal of Neuroscience Methods*, Vol.94, pp. 93-103,

Schlögl, A.& Supp, G. (2006). Analysing event-related EEG data with multivariate autoregressive parameters. In: *Progress in Brain Research*, Neuper & Klimesch (Eds), Vol. 159, pp. 135-147, Elsevier, Amsterdam, The Netherlands

Schmidt, R.A.& Lee, T.D. (1999). *Motor control and learning: a behavioral emphasis*. Human Kinetics, Champaign, IL

Schöner, G. (1994). Dynamic theory of action-perception patterns: The time-before-contact paradigm. *Human Movement Science*, Vol.13, pp. (415-439),

Schöner, G.& Kelso, J.A.S. (1988). A dynamic pattern theory of behavioral change. *Journal of Theoretical Biology*, Vol.135, pp. 501-524,

Singer, W. (1993). Synchronization of cortical activity and its putative role in information processing and learning. *Annual Review of Physiology*, Vol.55, pp. 349-374,

Stein, J. (1995). The posterior parietal cortex, the cerebellum and the visual guidance of movement. In: *Neural Control of Skilled Human Movement*, F.W.J. Cody (Ed). 31-49, The Physiological Society, London

Steriade, M., Gloor, P., Llinas, R.R., Lopes da Silva, F.H.& Mesulam, M.M. (1991). Basic mechanisms of cerebral rhythmic activities. *Electroencephalography and clinical Neurophysiology*, Vol.76, pp. 481-508,

Suffczynski, P., Pijn, P.J.M., Pfurtscheller, G.& Lopes da Silva, F.H. (1999). Event-related dynamics of alpha band rhythms: a neuronal network model of focal ERD/surround ERS. In: *Event-Related Desynchronization: Handbook of Electroencephalography and Clinical Neurophysiology*, G. Pfurtscheller & F.H. Lopes da Silva (Eds), Vol.6, 67-85, Elsevier, Amsterdam

Takahashi, D.Y., Baccalá, L.A.& Sameshima, K. (2008). Partial directed coherence asymptotics for VAR processes of infinite order. *International Journal of Bioelectromagnetism*, Vol.10, No.1, pp. 31-36,

Turvey, M.T.& Kugler, P.N. (1984). An ecological approach to perception and action. In: *Human Motor Actions: Bernstein Reassessed*, H.T.A. Whiting (Ed), 373-412, North-Holland, Amsterdam

Wang, G. & Takigawa, M. (1992). Directed coherence as a measure of interhemispheric correlation of EEG. *International Journal of Psychophysiology*, Vol. 13, pp. 119-128,

Warren, H.W. (1990). The perception-action coupling. In: *Sensory-Motor Organizations and Development in Infancy and Early Childhood*, H. Bloch & B.I. Bertenthal (Eds), 23-37, Kluwer Academic Pub., Netherlands

Westwood, D.A., Chapman, C.D.& Roy, E.A. (2000a). Pantomimed actions may be controlled by the ventral visual stream. *Experimental Brain Research*, Vol.130, pp. 545-548,

Westwood, D.A., Heath, M.& Roy, E.A. (2000b). The effect of a pictorial illusion on closed-loop and open-loop prehension. *Experimental Brain Research*, Vol.134, pp. 456-463,

Zaal, F.T.J.M., Bootsma, R.J., & van Wieringen, P.C. (1998). Coordination in prehension: Information-based coupling of reaching and grasping. *Experimental Brain Research*, Vol.119, pp. 427-435,

Zigmond, M.J., Bloom, F.E., Landis, S.C., Roberts, J.L.& Squire, L.R. (1999). *Fundamental Neuroscience*. Academic Press, San Diego, CA

# Chapter 2

# Electroencephalography (EEG) and Unconsciousness

Dongyu Wu and Ying Yuan

Additional information is available at the end of the chapter

http://dx.doi.org/10.5772/48346

## 1. Introduction

The commonest and simplest operational definition of consciousness is, the state of the patient's awareness of self and environment and his responsiveness to external stimulation and inner need. Therefore, unconsciousness has the opposite meaning, that is, a state of unawareness of self and environment or a suspension of those mental activities by which people are made aware of themselves and their environment, coupled with a diminished responsiveness to environmental stimuli. Loss of consciousness can have many different causes, for example, stroke, traumatic brain injury, anesthesia, brainstem lesions and sleep, the various causes of unconsciousness primarily interfering with different brain functions. Clinically, impaired consciousness such as coma, vegetative state (VS) and minimally conscious state (MCS) is a very common manifestation in subjects with acquired brain injury. Unconsciousness does not always consist of a general suppression of the entire activity of the central nervous system. Depending on the actual cause(s), many functions, such as protective reflexes and various cognitive processes, can remain intact. The Management of such a patient in VS or MCS requires carefully reaching the correct diagnosis, pronouncing an evidence-based prognosis, and thoughtfully considering the medical, ethical, and legal elements of optimum treatment (Bernat, 2006).

### 1.1. The anatomy and neurophysiology of unconsciousness

The pioneering studies of Moruzzi and Magoun in the 1940s showed that, electrical stimulation of the medial midbrain tegmentum and adjacent areas just above this level caused a lightly anesthetized animal to become suddenly alert and its EEG to change correspondingly, i.e., to become "desynchronized," in a manner identical to normal arousal by sensory stimuli. The sites at which stimulation led to arousal consisted of a series of points extending from the nonspecific medial thalamic nuclei down through the caudal midbrain. These points were situated along where anatomists had referred to as the reticular system or formation. Fibers from the reticular formation ascend to the thalamus and project to various nonspecific thalamic nuclei. From these nuclei, there is a diffuse distribution of connections to all parts of the cerebral cortex. This whole system is concerned with consciousness and is known as the ascending reticular activating system (ARAS). Moreover, sensory stimulation has a double effect—it conveys information to the brain from somatic structures and the environment and also activates those parts of the nervous system on which the maintenance of consciousness depends. The cerebral cortex not only receives impulses from the ascending reticular activating system but also modulates this incoming information via corticofugal projections to the reticular formation (Ropper and Brown, 2005). Intact consciousness requires normal functioning of the cortex of both cerebral hemispheres.

Consciousness can be divided into two main components: arousal (wakefulness and vigilance) and awareness (awareness of the environment and the self). Arousal is supported by several brainstem neuronal populations that directly project to both thalamic and subcortical neurons. Awareness is dependent upon the integrity of the cerebral cortex and its subcortical connections. Each of its many parts is located, to some extent, in anatomically defined regions of the brain (Zeman, 2001). Impairments of consciousness may thus be caused either by the simultaneous impairment of function of both cerebral hemispheres, or by damage to the reticular formation in the brainstem, and/or to its ascending projections (uncoupling of the cortex from the activating input of the reticular formation).

## 1.2. Clinical definition of unconsciousness

### *1.2.1. Coma*

Coma is a state of unresponsiveness in which the patient lies with the eyes closed, cannot be aroused, and has no awareness of self and surroundings. Coma may result from bilateral diffuse cortical or white matter damage or brainstem lesions bilaterally, affecting the subcortical reticular arousing systems, or from sudden large unilateral lesions that functionally disrupt the contralateral hemisphere. Coma is distinguished from syncope or concussion in terms of its duration, which is at least 1h. In general, comatose patients who survive begin to awaken and recover gradually within 2–4 weeks (Plum and Posner, 1983). Many factors such as etiology, age, the patient's general medical condition, clinical signs, and complementary examinations influence the management and prognosis of coma. Traumatic etiology is known to have a better outcome than non-traumatic anoxic cases.

### *1.2.2. Vegetative state*

Patients in a vegetative state (VS) are awake but are unaware of themselves or their environment. The VS is usually caused by diffuse lesions on the gray and white matter.

Characterized by 'wakefulness without awareness', patients regain their sleep–wake cycle, and may be aroused by painful or salient stimuli, but show no unambiguous signs of conscious perception or deliberate action, including communicative acts.

Persistent vegetative state (PVS) has been defined as a vegetative state remaining 1 month after acute traumatic or non-traumatic brain damage. It does not imply irreversibility. According to the Multi-Society Task Force on persistent vegetative state (PVS), the criteria for the diagnosis of VS are the following (1994): (1) no evidence of awareness of self or environment and an inability to interact with others; (2) no evidence of sustained, reproducible, purposeful, or voluntary behavioral responses to visual, auditory, tactile, or noxious stimuli; (3) no evidence of language comprehension or expression; (4) intermittent wakefulness manifested by the presence of sleep–wake cycles; (5) sufficiently preserved hypothalamic and brainstem autonomic functions to permit survival with medical and nursing care; (6) bowel and bladder incontinence; and (7) variably preserved cranial nerve and spinal reflexes. However, permanent vegetative state is irreversible. According to the Multi-Society Task Force on Permanent Vegetative State (1994), vegetative state may be regarded as permanent 3 months after non-traumatic brain damage or 12 months after traumatic injury. These guidelines are best applied to patients who have diffuse traumatic brain injuries and postanoxic events. Recovery from a vegetative state often occurs: younger age and a traumatic, rather than hypoxic–ischemic etiology.

### *1.2.3. Minimally conscious state*

According to Giacino's definition (Giacino et al. , 2002), the minimally conscious state (MCS) is a condition of severely altered consciousness in which limited but clearly discernible evidence of self or environmental awareness must be demonstrated on a reproducible or sustained basis by at least one of the following behaviors: (1) following simple commands; (2) gestural or verbal yes/no responses (regardless of accuracy); (3) intelligible verbalization; (4) purposeful behavior, including movements or affective behaviors that occur in contingent relation to relevant environmental stimuli and are not due to reflexive activity, such as, appropriate smiling or crying in response to the linguistic or visual content of emotional but not to neutral topics or stimuli; vocalizations or gestures that occur in direct response to the linguistic content of questions; reaching for objects that demonstrates a clear relationship between object location and direction of reach; touching or holding objects in a manner that accommodates the size and shape of the object; pursuit eye movement or sustained fixation that occurs in direct response to moving or salient stimuli.

Like the VS, the MCS may be chronic and sometimes permanent. Emergence from the MCS is defined by the ability to exhibit functional interactive communication or functional use of objects. Similar to the VS, traumatic etiology has a better prognosis than non-traumatic anoxic brain injuries. Preliminary data show that the overall outcome in the MCS is more favorable than in the VS (Giacino and Whyte, 2005, Laureys et al. , 2004a).

### *1.2.4. Brain death*

Most countries have published recommendations for the diagnosis of brain death but the diagnostic criteria differ from country to country. Some rely on the death of the brainstem only; others require death of the whole brain including the brainstem. However, the clinical assessments for brain death are the same and require the loss of all brainstem reflexes and the demonstration of continuing apnea in a persistently comatose patient (Laureys, Owen, 2004a). The central considerations in the diagnosis of brain death are: (1) absence of all cerebral functions; (2) absence of all brainstem functions, including spontaneous respiration; and (3) irreversibility of the state (Ropper and Brown, 2005). At present, no recovery from brain death has been reported.

### *1.2.5. Locked-in syndrome*

The locked-in syndrome (LIS), characterized by anarthria and quadriplegia with general preservation of cognition, must be distinguished from disorders of consciousness. The locked-in syndrome describes patients who are awake and conscious, but have no means of producing speech, limb, or facial movements, resembling patients in VS, and is most often caused by a lesion of the ventral pons (basis pontis) as a result of basilar artery occlusion. Locked-in syndrome is defined by sustained eye opening (bilateral ptosis should be ruled out as a complicating factor), awareness of the environment, aphonia or hypophonia, quadriplegia or quadriparesis, and vertical or lateral eye movement or blinking of the upper eyelid to signal yes/no responses (Giacino et al. , 1995). Eye or eyelid movements are the main method of communication. Since there is only motor output problem, LIS is not a disorder of consciousness (DOC).

Table 1 outlines the clinical features of disorders of consciousness and the locked-in syndrome.

## 1.3. Epidemiology of unconsciousness

Three categories of disorder can cause VS: acute traumatic and non-traumatic brain injuries; degenerative and metabolic brain disorders, and severe congenital malformations of the nervous system. However, the most common cause of VS and MCS is traumatic brain injury. Non-traumatic causes in adults include acute hypoxic-ischemic neuronal injury suffered during cardiopulmonary arrest, stroke, and meningoencephalitis (Tresch et al. , 1991). For children, causes of VS include trauma, meningitis, asphyxia, congenital malformations, and perinatal injuries (Ashwal et al. , 1992).

The Multi-society Task Force claimed that in the USA there are 10,000–25,000 adults and 4,000-10,000 children (about 56-140 per million) in a PVS (1994). This estimate was almost certainly high given that their prevalence model assumed that many patients with neurodegenerative diseases eventually progressed to a vegetative state and that many children were in a vegetative state from developmental malformations. According to an epidemiological survey of persistent vegetative state and minimally conscious state in

Austria, the point prevalence was 33.6 patients per million for VS and 15 per million for MCS in long-term care facilities (Donis and Kraftner, 2011). Without reliable epidemiologic measures, patients in MCS remain silent victims, unheard and uncounted.

| Clinical feature | Coma | Vegetative state | Minimally conscious state | Locked-in syndrome |
|---|---|---|---|---|
| **Consciousness** | None | None | Partial | Full |
| **Sleep/wake** | Absent | Present | Present | Present |
| **Motor function** | Reflex and postural responses only | Postures or withdraws to noxious stimuli<br>Occasional nonpurposeful movement | Localizes noxious stimuli<br>Reaches for objects<br>Holds or touches objects in a manner that accommodates size and shape<br>Automatic movements (e.g., scratching) | Quadriplegic |
| **Auditory function** | None | Startle<br>Brief orienting to sound | Localizes sound location<br>Inconsistent command following | Preserved |
| **Visual function** | None | Startle<br>Brief visual fixation | Sustained visual fixation<br>Sustained visual pursuit | Preserved |
| **Communication** | None | None | Contingent vocalization<br>Inconsistent but intelligible verbalization or gesture | Aphonic/Anarthric<br>Vertical eye movement and blinking usually intact |
| **Emotion** | None | None<br>Reflexive crying or smiling | Contingent smiling or crying | Preserved |

Quotes from Giacino JT, Ashwal S, Childs N, Cranford R, Jennett B, Katz DI, et al. The minimally conscious state: definition and diagnostic criteria. Neurology. 2002;58:349-53.

**Table 1.** Clinical features of disorders of consciousness and the locked-in syndrome

Patients with MCS may follow a survival time course distinguishable from other brain-injured patients. It has been suggested that patients in VS due to TBI have a lower mortality rate and longer survival compared with those with anoxia (Childs et al. , 1993). Survival in MCS depends on age; quality of care; comorbid illness and injury; and decisions to withhold or withdraw life-sustaining therapy. Survival estimates with severe brain injury are variable (Fins et al. , 2007). Young patients with MCS retain limited mobility and have longer life spans; 81% have an 8-year survival (Childs, Mercer, 1993).

## 2. Clinical assessment methods of unconsciousness

The assessment and prognosis of unconsciousness currently depends mainly on clinical scales and experience. The limitations of those scales are obvious. Subtle changes in levels of unconsciousness cannot be clearly and accurately captured, but depend greatly on the experience of the examiner (Stevens and Bhardwaj, 2006). Clinical commonly used scales of unconsciousness, such as the Glasgow Coma Scale (GCS), Rappaport Coma/Near-Coma Scale and JFK Coma Recovery Scale would be introduced as follows.

### 2.1. Glasgow Coma Scale (GCS)

The GCS is used to assess the level of consciousness after head injury and is now applicable to all acute medical and trauma patients. The scale comprises three tests: eye, verbal and motor responses. The three values separately as well as their sum are considered. The lowest possible GCS (the sum) is 3 (deep coma or death), while the highest is 15 (fully awake person).

The GCS, which was developed, validated, and used widely to assess the level of consciousness and prognosis of patients with acute traumatic brain injuries (Rowley and Fielding, 1991) and non-traumatic causes of coma (Mullie et al. , 1988), is insufficient for the assessment of vegetative state and minimally conscious state because of its crude measurement of awareness and its omission of relevant neurological functions (Howard and Hirsch, 1999).

| | | |
|---|---|---|
| **Eye Response** | Does not open eyes | 1 point |
| | Opens eyes in response to painful stimuli | 2 points |
| | Opens eyes in response to voice | 3 points |
| | Opens eyes spontaneously | 4 points |
| **Verbal Response** | Makes no sounds | 1 point |
| | Incomprehensible sounds | 2 points |
| | Utters inappropriate words | 3 points |
| | Confused, disoriented | 4 points |
| | Oriented, converses normally | 5 points |
| **Motor Response** | Makes no movements | 1 point |
| | Extension to painful stimuli (decerebrate response) | 2 points |
| | Abnormal flexion to painful stimuli (decorticate response) | 3 points |
| | Flexion / Withdrawal to painful stimuli | 4 points |
| | Localizes painful stimuli | 5 points |
| | Obeys commands | 6 points |

**Table 2.** Glasgow Coma Scale (GCS)

### 2.2. Rappaport coma/Near-coma scale

The Coma/Near Coma (CNC) scale was developed to measure small clinical changes in patients with severe brain injuries who function at very low levels characteristic of near-vegetative and vegetative states. The CNC was designed to provide reliable, valid, easy, and quick assessment of progress or lack of progress in low-level brain injured patients. The CNC has five levels, based on 11 items that can be scored to indicate severity of sensory, perceptual, and primitive response deficits. For the details, See *Rappaport, M. (2000). The Coma/Near Coma Scale. The Center for Outcome Measurement in Brain Injury. http://www.tbims.org/combi/cnc (accessed October 1, 2011).*

### 2.3. JFK Coma Recovery Scale-Revised

The JFK Coma Recovery Scale-Revised (CRS-R) comprises 6 subscales addressing auditory, visual, motor, oromotor/verbal, communication, and arousal processes. Scoring is based on the presence or absence of specific behavioral responses to sensory stimuli administered in a standardized manner. The lowest item on each subscale represents reflexive activity or no response, whereas the highest items represent cognitively mediated behaviors.

The CRS-R appears to meet minimal standards for measurement and evaluation tools designed for use in interdisciplinary medical rehabilitation. The scale can be administered reliably by trained examiners and produces reasonably stable scores over repeated assessments. Diagnostic application of the CRS-R suggests that the scale is capable of discriminating patients in an MCS from those in VS (Giacino et al. , 2004).

According to the report of a systematic review of behavioral assessment scales for disorders of consciousness (DOC), the CRS-R has excellent content validity and is the only scale to address all Aspen Workgroup criteria and may be used to assess DOC with minor reservations, while CNC may be used to assess DOC with major reservations (Seel et al. , 2010).

## 3. Functional neuroimaging and unconsciousness

Although bedside clinical assessment examination remains the criterion standard for establishing diagnosis in clinical practice, behavioral findings are often limited or ambiguous. Recently, the evidence from the non-invasive functional imaging techniques, especially functional magnetic resonance imaging (fMRI) and positron emission tomography (PET) provided clues to brain function in unconscious populations, suggests that some patients with DOC exhibit partially preserved conscious processing despite having no clinical or verbal output (Owen et al. , 2006) and may serve an adjunctive and useful information to the diagnosis and prognosis of these patients.

Recent advances in functional neuroimaging use so-called 'activation' studies to assess residual brain function in altered states of consciousness without the need for any overt response on the part of the patient. fMRI can capture precisely and visualize localized physiologic change in the brain induced by neuronal activity. Several fMRI and PET findings demonstrated that some MCS or VS patients retain islands of preserved cognitive, sensory and auditory function.

| | | |
|---|---|---|
| **Auditory Function Scale** | Consistent Movement to Command* | 4 |
| | Reproducible Movement to Command* | 3 |
| | Localization to Sound | 2 |
| | Auditory Startle | 1 |
| | None | 0 |
| **Visual Function Scale** | Object Recognition* | 5 |
| | Object Localization: Reaching* | 4 |
| | Visual Pursuit* | 3 |
| | Fixation* | 2 |
| | Visual Startle | 1 |
| | None | 0 |
| **Motor Function Scale** | Functional Object Use† | 6 |
| | Automatic Motor Response* | 5 |
| | Object Manipulation* | 4 |
| | Localization to Noxious Stimulation* | 3 |
| | Flexion Withdrawal | 2 |
| | Abnormal Posturing | 1 |
| | None/Flaccid | 0 |
| **Oromotor/Verbal Function Scale** | Intelligible Verbalization* | 3 |
| | Vocalization/Oral Movement | 2 |
| | Oral Reflexive Movement | 1 |
| | None | 0 |
| **Communication Scale** | Oriented† | 3 |
| | Functional: Accurate† | 2 |
| | Non-Functional: Intentional* | 1 |
| | None | 0 |
| **Arousal Scale** | Attention* | 3 |
| | Eye Opening without Stimulation | 2 |
| | Eye Opening with Stimulation | 1 |
| | Unarousable | 0 |

*Denotes MCS.
†Denotes emergence from MCS.

**Table 3.** JFK Coma Recovery Scale-Revised (CRS-R)

The VS patients show cortical activation limited to 'lower level' primary cortical areas. Noxious somatosensory stimulation, such as high-intensity electric stimulation of the median nerve at the wrist, induced activation of midbrain, contralateral thalamus, and primary somatosensory cortex. The somatosensory cortex was functionally disconnected from 'higher order' associative cortical areas, encompassing anterior cingulate, insular, prefrontal and posterior parietal cortices. In healthy controls, such stimuli activated primary and secondary somatosensory cortices, bilateral insular, posterior parietal and anterior cingulate cortices (Laureys et al. , 2002). In line with the results of the somatosensory activation study described above, the activated primary auditory cortex by auditory stimulation was also functionally disconnected from higher order areas encompassing posterior parietal, anterior cingulate and hippocampal areas, whereas in control subjects, stimuli activated bilateral primary and contralateral auditory association cortices (Boly et al. , 2004, Laureys et al. , 2000). Likewise, visual stimulation elicited activation in primary visual cortex (Giacino et al. , 2006). These studies support the view that simple somatosensory, auditory and visual stimuli typically activate primary cortices in patients with VS and fail to show robust activation in higher order associative cortices.

It is important to differentiate a patient in PVS from a patient in MCS, as the latter patient has a much higher chance of a favorable outcome. Some MCS patients may retain widely distributed cortical systems with potential for cognitive and sensory function, despite their inability to follow simple instructions or communicate reliably (Schiff et al. , 2005). PET and fMRI case reports incorporating complex auditory stimuli have shown large-scale network activation in the minimally conscious state that is not observed in unconscious vegetative patients (Bekinschtein et al. , 2005, Laureys et al. , 2004b).

However, it remains controversial whether the VS patients with atypical 'higher order' associative cortical activation have a good outcome. In some fMRI or/and PET studies, patients with higher-level associative cortical activation in VS progressed to MCS or recovered consciousness (Bekinschtein, Tiberti, 2005, Coleman et al. , 2007, Di et al. , 2007), which seem to show that atypical 'higher order' associative cortical activation in VS heralds recovery of some level of consciousness some months later. Other VS patients with 'higher level' associative cortical activation failed to subsequently recover (Staffen et al. , 2006), which was in line with the viewpoint that VS patients with atypical behavioral fragments can show residual isolated brain processing in the absence of clinical recovery (Schiff et al. , 2002) .

Functional connectivity of the brain, measured with fMRI techniques, seems to play a more important role for consciousness. Recently, the brain activity fluctuations in the default resting state have received increasing interest. The default mode network is defined as a set of areas encompassing the posterior-cingulate/precuneus, anterior cingulated/mesiofrontal cortex and temporo-parietal junctions, showing more activity at rest than during attention-demanding tasks. Some studies on resting state activity in DOC show that functional connectivity is disrupted in the task-negative or the default mode network. Cauda et al. studied three patients in a vegetative state, found the decreased connectivity in several brain regions, including the dorsolateral prefrontal cortex and anterior cingulated cortex, especially in the right hemisphere, the results showed a dysfunctional default mode network (Cauda et al. , 2009). Boly et al. demonstrated absent cortico-thalamic functional connectivity but partially preserved cortico-cortical connectivity within the default network in a vegetative state patient following cardio-respiratory arrest (Boly et al. , 2009). In this patient, anticorrelations could also be observed between the posterior cingulate/precuneus and a previously identified task-positive cortical network, but both correlations and anti-correlations were significantly reduced as compared to healthy controls. In the same study, a brain death patient studied two days after a massive cranial hemorrhage and evolution to a comatose state showed no residual functional connectivity (Boly, Tshibanda, 2009). In a more comprehensive study, fourteen non-communicative brain-damaged patients and fourteen healthy controls participated in a resting state fMRI protocol. Functional connectivity in all default network areas was found to be non-linearly correlated with the degree of consciousness, ranging from healthy volunteers and locked-in syndrome, to minimally conscious, vegetative and comatose patients. Furthermore, connectivity in the precuneus was found to be significantly stronger in MCS patients compared with VS patients, while locked-in syndrome patients' default network connectivity was shown to be not significantly different from that of healthy control subjects (Vanhaudenhuyse et al. , 2010).

Certainly, the two main approaches, hypothesis-driven seed-voxel and data-driven independent component analysis, employed in the analysis of resting state functional connectivity data present multiple methodological difficulties, especially in non-collaborative DOC patients. Improvements in motion artifact removal and spatial normalization are needed before fMRI resting state data can be used as proper biomarkers in severe brain injury.

In a word, we can only say functional imaging activation studies can provide valuable prognostic information, and future efforts should be needed.

## 4. Evoked potentials (EPs) and unconsciousness

### 4.1. Auditory evoked potentials (AEPs) and unconsciousness

Auditory evoked potentials (AEPs) can be used to trace the signal generated by a sound through the ascending auditory pathway. The evoked potential is generated in the cochlea, goes through the cochlear nerve, through the cochlear nucleus, superior olivary complex, lateral lemniscus, to the inferior colliculi in the midbrain, on to the medial geniculate body, and finally to the cortex. Brainstem auditory-evoked potentials (BAEPs) do not play a role in the prognosis for awakening, but only play a prognostic role in survival (Lew et al. , 2003, Young et al. , 2004).

A study of long-latency responses (LLRs) reported that a P300 component was observed in response to the patient's name in all patients with locked-in syndrome, in all MCS patients, and in 3 of 5 patients in VS. However, a P300 response does not necessarily reflect conscious perception and cannot be used to differentiate VS from MCS patients (Perrin et al. , 2006). Another study also demonstrated that MCS patients presented a larger P300 to the patient's own name, in the passive and in the active conditions. Moreover, the P300 to target stimuli was higher in the active than in the passive condition, suggesting voluntary compliance to task instructions like controls. In contrast, no P300s were observed for VS patients in response to their own name (Schnakers et al. , 2008). In conclusion, auditory LLRs are clinically useful for assessment of higher-order neural functions and processing in TBI patients. Auditory P300 protocols can be used to assess cognitive functions in this population (Folmer et al. , 2011).

Mismatch Negativity (MMN) is generated by the brain's automatic response to physical stimulus deviation from the preceding stimulus in repetitive auditory input, revealing that physical features of auditory stimuli are fully processed regardless whether they are attended to or not (Naatanen et al. , 2004). The auditory MMN (which can occur in response to deviance in pitch, intensity, or duration) is a fronto-central negative potential with primary generators in auditory cortex and a typical latency of 150–250ms after the onset of the deviant stimulus. Neural generators of the MMN might also include frontal cortex and thalamus (Naatanen et al. , 2007). Fischer et al. studied a series of 346 comatose patients and found that the presence of MMN is a predictor of awakening and precludes comatose patients from moving to a permanent vegetative state (Fischer et al. , 2004). Mismatch negativity has repeatedly shown to predict outcome after coma demonstrated that in the acute phase the presence of MMN predicted the exclusion of shifting into PVS. In the study of Kotchoubey et al., 6 months after the brain insult clinical improvement was observed more frequently in VS and MCS patients with a significant MMN than in those without the MMN (Kotchoubey et al. , 2005). Wijnen et al. recorded MMNs from 10 patients in VS every 2 weeks for an average period of 3.5 months and observed that with recovery to consciousness MMN-amplitudes increased and a sudden increase was seen in MMN amplitude when patients started to show inconsistent behavioral responses to simple commands. Thus, they concluded that MMN can be helpful in identifying the ability to recover from VS. Compared the prognostic value of MMN to auditory P300 elicited by the patient's own name, the use of novelty P3 elicited by the patient's name increases the prognostic value of MMN alone and improves the assessment of comatose patients by demonstrating the activation of higher-level cognitive functions (Fischer et al. , 2008). Moreover, a meta-analysis of Daltrozzo et al. indicated that MMN and P300 appeared to be reliable predictors of awakening in low-responsive patients with stroke or hemorrhage, trauma and metabolic encephalopathy etiologies (Daltrozzo et al. , 2007).

## 4.2. Somatosensory Evoked Potentials (SEPs) and unconsciousness

Somatosensory Evoked Potentials (SEPs) can trace the conduction of a sensory impulse (initiated by touch, painful stimuli, or mild electrical stimulation of the skin) from a patient's leg or wrist, through the limb and spinal column, and to record its arrival in contralateral somatosensory cortex. Short-latency somatosensory evoked potentials (SSEPs) refer to the primary response from the somatosensory cortex (S1).

Many studies have confirmed that the absence of cortical somatosensory-evoked potentials (SSEPs) such as N20 is good evidence to predict recovery from coma (Amantini et al. , 2005, Carter and Butt, 2005, Robinson et al. , 2003, Young, Wang, 2004). Lew et al. studied 22 patients who suffered severe TBI and observed that bilateral absence of median nerve SEP was strongly predictive of the worst functional outcome (Lew, Dikmen, 2003). However, these studies mainly focused on acute brain injury. Prolonged impaired consciousness (MCS and VS) have not been studied in such detail. Wu et al. studied 21 subjects in PVS and 16 in MCS and founded that SSEPs failed to distinguished subjects in PVS from those in MCS, which indicated that this measure might be limited in predicting outcome in this population (Wu et al. , 2011a).

## 5. EEG (traditional methods) and unconsciousness

Electroencephalography (EEG) can also provide a direct and dynamic measurement of electrical brain activity induced by neuronal functional activity in the cortex. EEG allows for an immediate examination of cortical or cortical–subcortical dysfunction in an inexpensive, safe, and readily available manner. It is an important tool in assessing unconscious patients.

### 5.1. Several scoring systems for grading the severity of EEG abnormalities

Changes in EEG patterns may indicate either deepening or lightening of coma, though orderly progression of coma through various EEG patterns does not always occur. Researchers have already agreed the following EEG patterns found after cardiac arrest are strongly associated with an poor neurologic outcome: generalized suppression; generalized burst–suppression; generalized periodic patterns, especially with epileptiform activity; and $\alpha$- or $\alpha$-/$\theta$-pattern coma (Young, 2000).

Synek developed one of the first EEG classification systems for comatose patients (Synek, 1988). Table 4 lists the Synek EEG Classification System. In his view, favorable outcome with survival seems to occur with both grade 1 and the "reactive type" of grade 2 abnormalities, with preservation of normal sleep features, and with frontal mono-rhythmic delta activity; prognostically uncertain patterns are "nonreactive" grade 2 abnormalities; diffuse delta activity with grade 3 abnormality, and the "reactive type of alpha pattern coma."; the following patterns are suggested to be prognostically malignant if persistent: grade 3 abnormality with small amplitude, diffuse, irregular delta activity; grade 4 ("burst suppression pattern"), in particular when epileptiform discharges are present and with "low-output EEG"; and grade 5 ("isoelectric EEG"); fatal outcome is also common with the "nonreactive type of alpha pattern coma" and the recently reported "theta pattern coma."

| Grade | Subgrade | Subsubgrade |
|---|---|---|
| **I (Regular alpha, some theta - reactive)** | | |
| **II (predominant theta)** | a. normal voltage, reactive<br>b. low voltage, nonreactive | |
| **III (delta/spindles)** | a. predominant delta, widespread, rhythmic, reactive<br>b. spindle coma<br>c. predominant delta, low voltage, irregular, nonreactive<br>d. predominant delta, medium voltage, usually nonreactive | |
| **IV (Burst suppression/alpha coma/theta coma/low voltage delta)** | a. burst suppression<br>b. alpha pattern coma<br>c. theta pattern coma<br>d. <20μV delta | (1) epileptiform activity<br>(2) no epileptiform activity<br>(1) some reactivity<br>(2) no reactivity |
| **V (Suppression)** | Electrocerebral silence (<2μV) | |

**Table 4.** Synek (1988) EEG Classification System

Young et al. suggested a revised EEG Classification System (Young et al. , 1997). Table 5 lists the Young EEG Classification System. This system for classifying EEGs in comatose patients has a higher inter-observer reliability than the Synek's.

| Category | Subcategory |
|---|---|
| **I Delta/theta > 50% of recording (not theta coma)** | (1) Reactivity<br>(2) No reactivity |
| **II Triphasic waves** | |
| **III Burst-suppression** | (1) With epileptiform activity<br>(2)Without epileptiform activity |
| **IV Alpha/theta/spindle coma (unreactive)** | |
| **V Epileptiform activity (not in burst-suppression pattern)** | (1) Generalized<br>(2) Focal or multifocal |
| **VI Suppression** | (1) <20μV, but > 10μV<br>(2) ≤10μV |
| **Guideline:**<br>**1. Burst-suppression pattern should have generalized flattening at standard sensitivity for ≥ 1 second at least every 20 seconds.**<br>**2. Suppression: for this category, voltage criteria should be met for the entire record; there should be no reactivity.**<br>**3. When > 1 category applies, select the most critical:**<br>**• Suppression is the most serious category.**<br>**• Burst-suppression pattern is more important than the category of triphasic waves which is more significant than dysrhythmia or delta.**<br>**• Alpha pattern coma is more important than focal spikes, triphasic waves, dysrhythmia or delta categories.** | |

**Table 5.** Young (1997) EEG Classification System

Husain presented a review of the EEG patterns commonly seen in coma (Husain, 2006). In this review, the author suggested that intermittent rhythmic delta activity (IRDA, consisting of 2 to 3 Hz sinusoidal waves occurring in a rhythmic but intermittent manner), triphasic waves (TW, blunt, delta (2 to 3 Hz) waves which consist of a high-voltage positive wave preceded and followed by lower amplitude negative waves) are seen in lighter stages of coma; continuous high-voltage delta activity has a poorer outcome than IRDA and TW; periodic lateralized epileptiform discharges (PLEDs), the prognosis depends on their etiology: those related to seizures often have a favorable outcome, whereas those due to infection and stroke have a more variable prognosis; generalized periodic epileptiform discharges (GPEDs), the prognosis depends on their etiology: if the GPEDs are due to medication overdose, outcome may be good, whereas the etiology is anoxia, outcome is usually poor; burst-suppression (generalized, synchronous bursts of high-voltage, mixed-frequency activity alternating with periods of suppression of EEG activity), prognosis is greatly dependent on etiology: patients manifesting this pattern after cardiac arrest are likely to have a much worse outcome; Low-voltage, slow, non-reactive EEG (the predominant activity is of theta and delta frequencies and the amplitude is less than 20μV) and electrocerebral inactivity (ECI), the prognosis is poor; spindle coma, the prognosis is often favorable; alpha coma, the etiology due to cardiorespiratory arrest is poor, due to toxic encephalopathy is favorable, and due to locked-in syndrome is poor; beta coma, the most common cause for beta coma is overdose of sedative-hypnotic medications and the prognosis is usually favorable.

### 5.2. Quantitative EEG and unconsciousness

Signal processing and computer technology have enabled the quantification of conventional electroencephalogram (EEG) findings. Digital EEG is paperless recording, storage and display with many advantages over traditional paper recordings. Quantitative EEG (QEEG) is any mathematical or statistical analysis along with the various graphical displays made from digital EEG. The most commonly used method is frequency spectrum analysis based on fast Fourier transform.

Most subjects in VS have profound generalized slowing of background activity with delta rhythms that do not react to stimuli; subjects with the most severe forms of VS show electrocerebral silence (Bernat, 2006). Most subjects in MCS show diffuse slowing in the theta or delta range (Giacino and Whyte, 2005), or in the theta or slow alpha (7.5–8 Hz) range (Fingelkurts et al., 2012, Kotchoubey, Lang, 2005). Since the spectrum of EEG malignant categories (suppression, burst-suppression, alpha and theta coma, and generalized periodic complexes combined) is greatly variable (Young, 2000), it is difficult to quantify different EEG features of malignant categories. Certain EEG features are associated with a poor outcome and, in some cases, useful in predicting eventual survival. However, the predictive value of individual classifications has not been adequately addressed (Husain, 2006, Young, 2000).

### 5.3. Other EEG analytical methods and unconsciousness

Other QEEG techniques include: monitoring and trending, source analysis, coherence analysis, EEG brain maps, et al. Coherence analysis, defined as a statistical measure of cross-correlation between two EEG signals in the frequency domain, and associated with functional coupling, is another commonly used method. Kane et al. investigated the relationship between quantitative EEG and BAEP measures and outcome, in 60 comatose patients after severe, closed head injury and the result indicated that there was regional information in EEG power spectra over the left hemisphere, which could be used in prognostic predictions for patients in coma after severe TBI (Kane et al. , 1998). Leon-Carrion et al. studied 7 MCS patients and 9 patients with severe neurocognitive disorders and the results stressed the importance of fronto-temporal-parietal associative cortices within the "awareness-regions" model and also suggest a relation between excess of slow wave activity and diminished level of awareness in brain injury population (Leon-Carrion et al. , 2008).

## 6. Nonlinear dynamics analysis (NDA) and unconsciousness

During the past two decades, nonlinear dynamics analysis (NDA) has become a common way to study neural mechanisms underlying cognition. The EEG is complex and of limited predictability because its ultra-high-dimensional nature makes it in essence a stochastic system (Jansen, 1991, Pritchard and Duke, 1995). NDA can characterize the dynamics of the neural networks underlying the EEG (Jelles et al. , 1999). Thus, it is suggested that NDA provides a useful tool for studying dynamic changes and abstracting correlations within cortical networks, such as the degree of synchronization within local neural networks and the coupling between distant cortical neural networks. NDA is derived from the mathematical theory of nonlinear dynamical systems. NDA has demonstrated that the decreased complexity of EEG patterns and reduced functional connections in the cerebral cortex likely are due to decreased nonlinear cell-dynamics as well as linear and nonlinear couplings between cortical areas (Jeong, 2004).

## 6.1. Principles of different NDA methods

### *6.1.1. Lempel-Ziv complexity (LZC)*

Lempel and Ziv proposed a useful complexity measure that characterizes degrees of order in and development of spatiotemporal patterns. Lempel-Ziv complexity (LZC) quantifies the complexity of time series and is well suited to the analysis of non-stationary biomedical signals of short length. Several studies showed that C(n) (a nonlinear index of complexity) is a useful and promising EEG-derived parameter for characterizing the depth of anesthesia (Zhang et al. , 2001).

LZC analysis is based upon a coarse-graining of the measurements, such that the EEG time series must be transformed into a finite symbol sequence. To do this, we used a simple binary sequence conversion (zeros and ones): Data values below or equal the mean of the given sequence were assigned the symbol "0," and the values above the mean were assigned the symbol "1". This algorithm gives the number of distinct patterns contained in the given finite sequence S=s1, s2, …, sn.

Once digitized, the EEG sequences were scanned according to the method of Kaspar and Schuster (Kaspar and Schuster, 1987). The corresponding complexity measure, c(n) increased by 1 unit when a new subsequence pattern was found in the process, and the next symbol was regarded as the beginning of the next subsequence pattern. The pattern searching continued until the last symbol was scanned. For instance, a time series of EEG signal (6.65, 2.63, 7.15, 1.04, 1.68, 5.55, 3.67, 4.51,… ) whose average was 4.11 could be converted into a binary sequence, 10100101…; c(n) of the binary sequence was 4, since different patterns observed in it were 1, 0, 100 and 101. More details of the LZC calculation can be found in the literature (Kaspar and Schuster, 1987, Zhang, Roy, 2001).

In order to obtain a complexity measure that is independent of the sequence length, c(n) was normalized. For a binary conversion, Lempel and Ziv (Lempel and Ziv, 1976) demonstrated that:

$$\lim_{n\to\infty} c(n) = b(n) \equiv \frac{n}{\log_2(n)}$$

such that c(n) could be normalized via b(n):

$$LZC = \frac{c(n)}{b(n)}$$

LZC usually ranges between zero and one. It is a nonlinear dynamic measure indicating the rate of appearance of the new patterns in a time series. A larger LZC implies a greater chance of the occurrence of new sequence patterns and thus a more complex dynamical behavior (Li et al. , 2008). LZC can be viewed as independent of number of samples when n is large (Zhang, Roy, 2001).

In Fig. 1, we present the four LZC analysis steps. The first step consisted in a pre-processing of the signals: artifact-free epoch selection and band-pass filtering. In the second step, the EEG data was transformed into a binary sequence through so-called coarse-graining procedure. The third step was subsequence pattern finding, used to estimate the complexity of the binary sequence – c(n). Finally, the normalized LZ complexity of the signals was calculated.

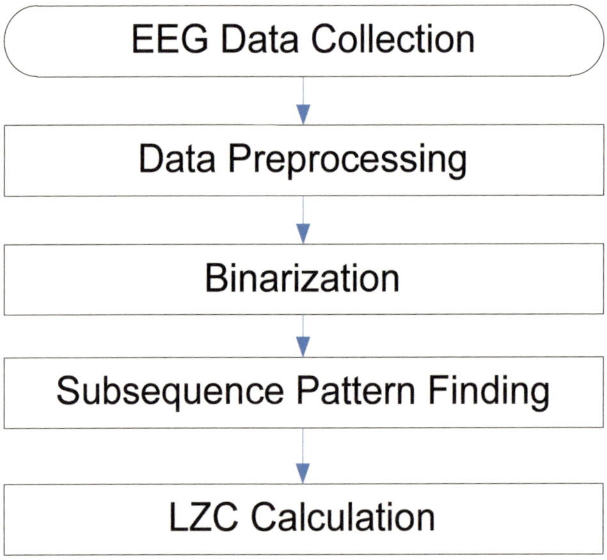


**Figure 1.** Block diagram of the steps followed in the LZC analysis: signal pre-processing, binarization, subsequence pattern finding and LZC calculation.

### *6.1.2. Approximate entropy (ApEn)*

Entropy, when considered as a physical concept, is related to the amount of "disorder" in the system. Approximate entropy can quantify the irregularity of data time series, i.e., the predictability of subsequent amplitude values based upon the knowledge of the previous amplitude values. Entropy of the EEG measures the regularity of the signal: high levels of entropy during anesthesia demonstrate that the subject is awake, whereas low levels of entropy correlate with deeper unconsciousness (Anderson et al. , 2004, Bruhn et al. , 2003, Hans et al. , 2005, Vakkuri et al. , 2004).

Approximate entropy is a measure of system complexity that was proposed by Pincus and Singer (Pincus and Singer, 1996). It is computed as follows:

$$ApEn(m,r,N) = \lim_{N\to\infty}[\phi^m(r) - \phi^{m+1}(r)]$$

$$\phi^m(r) = \frac{1}{N-m+1}\sum_{i=1}^{N-m+1} \ln C_i^m(r)$$

where C is the correlation integral.

The absolute value of approximate entropy is influenced by three parameters: the length of the epoch (N), the number of previous values used for the prediction of the subsequent value (m), and a filtering level (r). The noise filter defines the tolerance r that discerns "close" and "not close" subvectors of length "N." "r" measures the amount of noise in the data that is filtered out in the ensuing calculation.

ApEn calibrates an extent of serial interrelationships, quantifying a continuum that ranges from totally ordered (zero) to completely random (infinite). It assigns a non-negative number to a time series, with larger values corresponding to more complexity or irregularity in the data (Pincus, 2001). With increasing irregularity, knowing past values will not enable reliable prediction of future values, and approximate entropy will increase. Thus, decreasing irregularity (decreased ApEn) will cause lowered complexity in the time series, i.e. reduced nonlinear cell-dynamics or interaction of cortical networks.

### 6.1.3. *Cross aproximate entropy (C-ApEn)*

Cross approximate entropy (C-ApEn) measures the degree of dissimilarity between two concurrent series. A thematically similar quantification of two-variable asynchrony can aid in uncovering subtle disruptions in complicated network dynamics (Pincus, 2006). It is a recently introduced technique for analyzing two related time series to measure the degree of their asynchrony. C-ApEn is very similar to ApEn in design and intent, differing only in that it compares sequences from one series with those of the second (Richman and Moorman, 2000).

Given two time series of N points,

$$\{u(j); 1 \le j \le N\} \quad \text{and} \quad \{v(j); 1 \le j \le N\}$$

form the vectors

$$x_m(i) = \{u(i+k) : 0 \le k \le m-1\}$$
$$y_m(i) = \{v(i+k) : 0 \le k \le m-1\}$$

in which, u and v are the time series, m is the dimension of the vector, r is the same threshold used in the definition of ApEn, and N is the length of the time series. The distance between two such vectors is defined:

$$d[x_m(i), y_m(j)] = \max\{[u(i+k) - v(j+k)] : 0 \le k \le m-1\}$$

$C_i^m(r)(v \| u)$ is defined as the number of $y_m(j)$ within r of $x_m(i)$ divided by N-m+1, such that

$$\phi^m(r)(v \| u) = \frac{1}{N-m+1} \sum_{i=1}^{N-m+1} \ln\left[C_i^m(r)(v \| u)\right]$$

Lastly, the estimated approximate entropy of finite series is:

$$Cross - ApEn(m,r,N)(v \| u) = \phi^m(r)(v \| u) - \phi^{m+1}(r)(v \| u)$$

While the single-channel ApEn measures the temporal complexity of the EEG, the two-channel C-ApEn reflects the spatial decorrelation of cortical potentials from two remote sites (Hudetz, 2002). Since conscious cognitive processes depend on functional brain regions networks, C-ApEn could reflect the general state of functional connectivity of the brain that supports conscious processes.

What does raised C-ApEn mean about inter-cortical functional connectivity? This question is of great importance. According to Hudetz and Sleigh's explanation, EEG entropy should not be viewed simply as an indicator of disorder, but as a measure of the number of possible microstates a cortical neuronal network may access. The greater the number of microstates, the higher the informational content they represent (Hudetz, 2002, Sleigh et al. , 2001). Therefore, C-ApEn may be interpreted as a measure of the number of states independently accessible by the two cortical areas. Thus, an increase in C-ApEn during painful or auditory stimuli may indicate not only an increase in the number of independent microstates available for the two cortical areas, but also increased inter-cortical communication or information flow (Wu et al. , 2011b).

### 6.2. Clinical application of NDA correlated with unconsciousness

NDA also can quantify the depth of anesthesia and sedation, and has been shown to be a sensitive and agent-specific correlate of the central effects of anesthetics. Researchers have demonstrated that LZC and ApEn can distinguish between awake and anaesthetized state of human subjects (Anderson, Barr, 2004, Bruhn, Bouillon, 2003, Ferenets et al. , 2006, Ferenets et al. , 2007, Hans, Dewandre, 2005, Kumar et al. , 2007, Noh et al. , 2006, Vakkuri, Yli-Hankala, 2004, Voss et al. , 2006, Zhang, Roy, 2001). In sleep research ApEn was statistically significantly lower during Stage IV and higher during wake and REM sleep (Burioka et al. , 2005, Papadelis et al. , 2007).

### 6.3. Application of NDA in assessing unconsciousness

Wu et al. studied 21 patients in PVS, 16 in MCS and 30 normal conscious subjects (control group) with brain trauma or stroke. EEG was recorded under three conditions: eyes closed, auditory stimuli and painful stimuli. EEG nonlinear indices such as Lempel-Ziv complexity (LZC), approximate entropy (ApEn) and cross-approximate entropy (C-ApEn) were calculated for all subjects. The results showed that the PVS subjects had the lowest nonlinear indices, followed by the MCS subjects, and the control group had the highest; the PVS and MCS group had poorer response to auditory and painful stimuli than the control group; Under painful stimuli, nonlinear indices of subjects who recovered (REC) increased more significantly than non-REC subjects. The author considered that with EEG nonlinear analysis, the degree of suppression for PVS and MCS could be quantified and the changes of brain function for unconscious subjects could be captured by NDA. The possible mechanism might be that recovery of unconsciousness and the degree of suppression of unconsciousness are mediated through the brain cortex; NDA can reflect different levels of consciousness by measuring the complexity of the neuron networks in the brain cortex (Wu, Cai, 2011a).

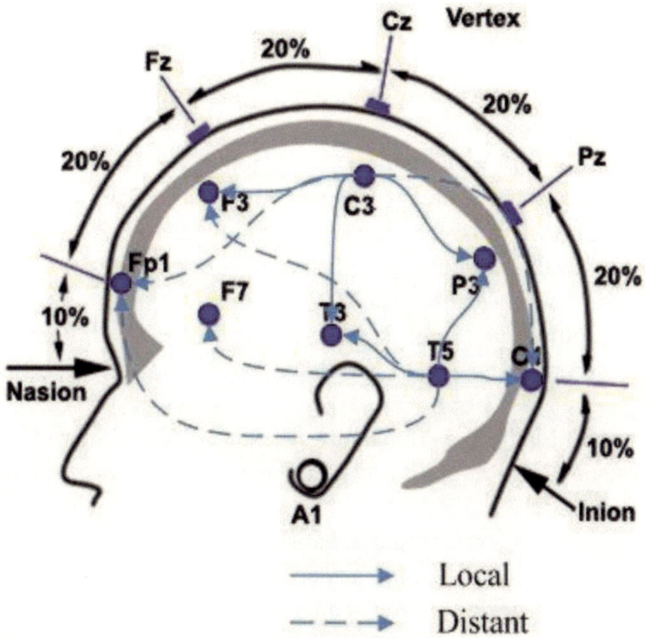


**Figure 2.** Schematic diagram of local and distant C-ApEn pairs.

Further study with C-ApEn was carried out to investigate the cortical response to painful and auditory stimuli for subjects in PVS and MCS, and measure the interconnection of the residual cortical functional islands. The results showed that interconnection of local and distant cortical networks of patients in PVS was generally suppressed, and painful or auditory stimulation could hardly cause any activation of associative cortices; instead, interconnection of local cortical networks of patients in MCS improved significantly; the only significant difference with the normal conscious subjects existed in the unaffected distant cortical networks. The author also present some question: does raised C-ApEn of patients in VS and MCS under various stimulation conditions mean a better prognosis? Could C-ApEn be used as a feedback index of such resuscitation therapies as repetitive transcranial magnetic stimulation (rTMS) and transcranial direct current stimulation (tDCS) that could increase the excitability of cortical regions of interest? Further research is needed to answer these questions (Wu, Cai, 2011b).

## Author details

Dongyu Wu* and Ying Yuan
*Department of Rehabilitation, Xuanwu Hospital of Capital Medical University, Xicheng District, Beijing, China*

## Acknowledgement

This chapter was supported by two grants from National Natural Science Foundation of China (Grant Nos. 30600186 and 81171011).

## 7. References

Medical aspects of the persistent vegetative state (1). The Multi-Society Task Force on PVS. N Engl J Med. 1994;330:1499-508.

Amantini A, Grippo A, Fossi S, Cesaretti C, Piccioli A, Peris A, et al. Prediction of 'awakening' and outcome in prolonged acute coma from severe traumatic brain injury: evidence for validity of short latency SEPs. Clin Neurophysiol. 2005;116:229-35.

Anderson RE, Barr G, Owall A, Jakobsson J. Entropy during propofol hypnosis, including an episode of wakefulness. Anaesthesia. 2004;59:52-6.

Ashwal S, Bale JF, Jr., Coulter DL, Eiben R, Garg BP, Hill A, et al. The persistent vegetative state in children: report of the Child Neurology Society Ethics Committee. Ann Neurol. 1992;32:570-6.

Bekinschtein T, Tiberti C, Niklison J, Tamashiro M, Ron M, Carpintiero S, et al. Assessing level of consciousness and cognitive changes from vegetative state to full recovery. Neuropsychol Rehabil. 2005;15:307-22.

Bernat JL. Chronic disorders of consciousness. Lancet. 2006;367:1181-92.

Boly M, Faymonville ME, Peigneux P, Lambermont B, Damas P, Del Fiore G, et al. Auditory processing in severely brain injured patients: differences between the minimally conscious state and the persistent vegetative state. Arch Neurol. 2004;61:233-8.

Boly M, Tshibanda L, Vanhaudenhuyse A, Noirhomme Q, Schnakers C, Ledoux D, et al. Functional connectivity in the default network during resting state is preserved in a vegetative but not in a brain dead patient. Human brain mapping. 2009;30:2393-400.

Bruhn J, Bouillon TW, Radulescu L, Hoeft A, Bertaccini E, Shafer SL. Correlation of approximate entropy, bispectral index, and spectral edge frequency 95 (SEF95) with clinical signs of "anesthetic depth" during coadministration of propofol and remifentanil. Anesthesiology. 2003;98:621-7.

Burioka N, Miyata M, Cornelissen G, Halberg F, Takeshima T, Kaplan DT, et al. Approximate entropy in the electroencephalogram during wake and sleep. Clin EEG Neurosci. 2005;36:21-4.

Carter BG, Butt W. A prospective study of outcome predictors after severe brain injury in children. Intensive Care Med. 2005;31:840-5.

---

* Corresponding Author

Cauda F, Micon BM, Sacco K, Duca S, D'Agata F, Geminiani G, et al. Disrupted intrinsic functional connectivity in the vegetative state. J Neurol Neurosurg Psychiatry. 2009;80:429-31.

Childs NL, Mercer WN, Childs HW. Accuracy of diagnosis of persistent vegetative state. Neurology. 1993;43:1465-7.

Coleman MR, Rodd JM, Davis MH, Johnsrude IS, Menon DK, Pickard JD, et al. Do vegetative patients retain aspects of language comprehension? Evidence from fMRI. Brain. 2007;130:2494-507.

Daltrozzo J, Wioland N, Mutschler V, Kotchoubey B. Predicting coma and other low responsive patients outcome using event-related brain potentials: a meta-analysis. Clin Neurophysiol. 2007;118:606-14.

Di HB, Yu SM, Weng XC, Laureys S, Yu D, Li JQ, et al. Cerebral response to patient's own name in the vegetative and minimally conscious states. Neurology. 2007;68:895-9.

Donis J, Kraftner B. The prevalence of patients in a vegetative state and minimally conscious state in nursing homes in Austria. Brain injury : [BI]. 2011;25:1101-7.

Ferenets R, Lipping T, Anier A, Jantti V, Melto S, Hovilehto S. Comparison of entropy and complexity measures for the assessment of depth of sedation. IEEE Trans Biomed Eng. 2006;53:1067-77.

Ferenets R, Vanluchene A, Lipping T, Heyse B, Struys MM. Behavior of entropy/complexity measures of the electroencephalogram during propofol-induced sedation: dose-dependent effects of remifentanil. Anesthesiology. 2007;106:696-706.

Fingelkurts AA, Bagnato S, Boccagni C, Galardi G. EEG oscillatory states as neuro-phenomenology of consciousness as revealed from patients in vegetative and minimally conscious states. Consciousness and cognition. 2012;21:149-69.

Fins JJ, Master MG, Gerber LM, Giacino JT. The minimally conscious state: a diagnosis in search of an epidemiology. Arch Neurol. 2007;64:1400-5.

Fischer C, Dailler F, Morlet D. Novelty P3 elicited by the subject's own name in comatose patients. Clin Neurophysiol. 2008;119:2224-30.

Fischer C, Luaute J, Adeleine P, Morlet D. Predictive value of sensory and cognitive evoked potentials for awakening from coma. Neurology. 2004;63:669-73.

Folmer RL, Billings CJ, Diedesch-Rouse AC, Gallun FJ, Lew HL. Electrophysiological assessments of cognition and sensory processing in TBI: applications for diagnosis, prognosis and rehabilitation. International journal of psychophysiology : official journal of the International Organization of Psychophysiology. 2011;82:4-15.

Giacino J, Whyte J. The vegetative and minimally conscious states: current knowledge and remaining questions. J Head Trauma Rehabil. 2005;20:30-50.

Giacino JT, Ashwal S, Childs N, Cranford R, Jennett B, Katz DI, et al. The minimally conscious state: definition and diagnostic criteria. Neurology. 2002;58:349-53.

Giacino JT, Hirsch J, Schiff N, Laureys S. Functional neuroimaging applications for assessment and rehabilitation planning in patients with disorders of consciousness. Arch Phys Med Rehabil. 2006;87:S67-76.

Giacino JT, Kalmar K, Whyte J. The JFK Coma Recovery Scale-Revised: measurement characteristics and diagnostic utility. Arch Phys Med Rehabil. 2004;85:2020-9.

Giacino JT, Zasler ND, Whyte J, Katz DI, Glen M, Andary M. Recommendations for Use of Uniform Nomenclature Pertinent to Patients with Severe Alterations in Consciousness. Arch Phys Med Rehab. 1995;76:205-9.

Hans P, Dewandre PY, Brichant JF, Bonhomme V. Comparative effects of ketamine on Bispectral Index and spectral entropy of the electroencephalogram under sevoflurane anaesthesia. Br J Anaesth. 2005;94:336-40.

Howard R, Hirsch N. Coma, vegetative state, and locked-in syndrome. In: Miller D, Raps E, editors. Critical care neurology. Boston: Butterworth-Heinemann; 1999. p. 91-120.

Hudetz AG. Effect of volatile anesthetics on interhemispheric EEG cross-approximate entropy in the rat. Brain Res. 2002;954:123-31.

Husain AM. Electroencephalographic assessment of coma. J Clin Neurophysiol. 2006;23:208-20.

Jansen BH. Quantitative analysis of electroencephalograms: is there chaos in the future? Int J Biomed Comput. 1991;27:95-123.

Jelles B, Strijers RL, Hooijer C, Jonker C, Stam CJ, Jonkman EJ. Nonlinear EEG analysis in early Alzheimer's disease. Acta Neurol Scand. 1999;100:360-8.

Jeong J. EEG dynamics in patients with Alzheimer's disease. Clin Neurophysiol. 2004;115:1490-505.

Kane NM, Moss TH, Curry SH, Butler SR. Quantitative electroencephalographic evaluation of non-fatal and fatal traumatic coma. Electroencephalogr Clin Neurophysiol. 1998;106:244-50.

Kaspar F, Schuster HG. Easily calculable measure for the complexity of spatiotemporal patterns. Phys Rev A. 1987;36:842-8.

Kotchoubey B, Lang S, Mezger G, Schmalohr D, Schneck M, Semmler A, et al. Information processing in severe disorders of consciousness: vegetative state and minimally conscious state. Clin Neurophysiol. 2005;116:2441-53.

Kumar A, Anand S, Chari P, Yaddanapudi LN, Srivastava A. A set of EEG parameters to predict clinically anaesthetized state in humans for halothane anaesthesia. J Med Eng Technol. 2007;31:46-53.

Laureys S, Faymonville ME, Degueldre C, Fiore GD, Damas P, Lambermont B, et al. Auditory processing in the vegetative state. Brain. 2000;123 ( Pt 8):1589-601.

Laureys S, Faymonville ME, Peigneux P, Damas P, Lambermont B, Del Fiore G, et al. Cortical processing of noxious somatosensory stimuli in the persistent vegetative state. Neuroimage. 2002;17:732-41.

Laureys S, Owen AM, Schiff ND. Brain function in coma, vegetative state, and related disorders. Lancet Neurol. 2004a;3:537-46.

Laureys S, Perrin F, Faymonville ME, Schnakers C, Boly M, Bartsch V, et al. Cerebral processing in the minimally conscious state. Neurology. 2004b;63:916-8.

Lempel A, Ziv J. On the complexity of finite sequences. IEEE Trans Inform Theor. 1976;22:75-81.

Leon-Carrion J, Martin-Rodriguez JF, Damas-Lopez J, Barroso y Martin JM, Dominguez-Morales MR. Brain function in the minimally conscious state: a quantitative neurophysiological study. Clin Neurophysiol. 2008;119:1506-14.

Lew HL, Dikmen S, Slimp J, Temkin N, Lee EH, Newell D, et al. Use of somatosensory-evoked potentials and cognitive event-related potentials in predicting outcomes of patients with severe traumatic brain injury. Am J Phys Med Rehabil. 2003;82:53-61; quiz 2-4, 80.

Li Y, Tong S, Liu D, Gai Y, Wang X, Wang J, et al. Abnormal EEG complexity in patients with schizophrenia and depression. Clin Neurophysiol. 2008;119:1232-41.

Mullie A, Verstringe P, Buylaert W, Houbrechts H, Michem N, Delooz H, et al. Predictive value of Glasgow coma score for awakening after out-of-hospital cardiac arrest. Cerebral Resuscitation Study Group of the Belgian Society for Intensive Care. Lancet. 1988;1:137-40.

Naatanen R, Paavilainen P, Rinne T, Alho K. The mismatch negativity (MMN) in basic research of central auditory processing: a review. Clin Neurophysiol. 2007;118:2544-90.

Naatanen R, Pakarinen S, Rinne T, Takegata R. The mismatch negativity (MMN): towards the optimal paradigm. Clin Neurophysiol. 2004;115:140-4.

Noh GJ, Kim KM, Jeong YB, Jeong SW, Yoon HS, Jeong SM, et al. Electroencephalographic approximate entropy changes in healthy volunteers during remifentanil infusion. Anesthesiology. 2006;104:921-32.

Owen AM, Coleman MR, Boly M, Davis MH, Laureys S, Pickard JD. Detecting awareness in the vegetative state. Science. 2006;313:1402.

Papadelis C, Chen Z, Kourtidou-Papadeli C, Bamidis PD, Chouvarda I, Bekiaris E, et al. Monitoring sleepiness with on-board electrophysiological recordings for preventing sleep-deprived traffic accidents. Clin Neurophysiol. 2007;118:1906-22.

Perrin F, Schnakers C, Schabus M, Degueldre C, Goldman S, Bredart S, et al. Brain response to one's own name in vegetative state, minimally conscious state, and locked-in syndrome. Arch Neurol. 2006;63:562-9.

Pincus S, Singer BH. Randomness and degrees of irregularity. Proc Natl Acad Sci U S A. 1996;93:2083-8.

Pincus SM. Assessing serial irregularity and its implications for health. Ann N Y Acad Sci. 2001;954:245-67.

Pincus SM. Approximate entropy as a measure of irregularity for psychiatric serial metrics. Bipolar Disord. 2006;8:430-40.

Plum F, Posner J. The diagnosis of stupor and coma. 3rd ed. Philadelphia: FA Davis; 1983.

Pritchard WS, Duke DW. Measuring "chaos" in the brain: a tutorial review of EEG dimension estimation. Brain Cogn. 1995;27:353-97.

Richman JS, Moorman JR. Physiological time-series analysis using approximate entropy and sample entropy. Am J Physiol Heart Circ Physiol. 2000;278:H2039-49.

Robinson LR, Micklesen PJ, Tirschwell DL, Lew HL. Predictive value of somatosensory evoked potentials for awakening from coma. Crit Care Med. 2003;31:960-7.

Ropper A, Brown R. Coma and related disorders of consciousness In: Ropper A, Samuels M, editors. Adams & Victor's Principles of Neurology. 8th ed. New York: McGraw-Hill; 2005. p. 302-21.

Rowley G, Fielding K. Reliability and accuracy of the Glasgow Coma Scale with experienced and inexperienced users. Lancet. 1991;337:535-8.

Schiff ND, Ribary U, Moreno DR, Beattie B, Kronberg E, Blasberg R, et al. Residual cerebral activity and behavioural fragments can remain in the persistently vegetative brain. Brain. 2002;125:1210-34.

Schiff ND, Rodriguez-Moreno D, Kamal A, Kim KH, Giacino JT, Plum F, et al. fMRI reveals large-scale network activation in minimally conscious patients. Neurology. 2005;64:514-23.

Schnakers C, Perrin F, Schabus M, Majerus S, Ledoux D, Damas P, et al. Voluntary brain processing in disorders of consciousness. Neurology. 2008;71:1614-20.

Seel RT, Sherer M, Whyte J, Katz DI, Giacino JT, Rosenbaum AM, et al. Assessment scales for disorders of consciousness: evidence-based recommendations for clinical practice and research. Arch Phys Med Rehabil. 2010;91:1795-813.

Sleigh JW, Olofsen E, Dahan A, de Goede J, Steyn-Rosser A. Entropies of the EEG: the effects of general anaesthesia. Proceedings of the Fifth International Conference on Memory, Awareness and Consciousness. USA2001.

Staffen W, Kronbichler M, Aichhorn M, Mair A, Ladurner G. Selective brain activity in response to one's own name in the persistent vegetative state. J Neurol Neurosurg Psychiatry. 2006;77:1383-4.

Stevens RD, Bhardwaj A. Approach to the comatose patient. Crit Care Med. 2006;34:31-41.

Synek VM. Prognostically important EEG coma patterns in diffuse anoxic and traumatic encephalopathies in adults. J Clin Neurophysiol. 1988;5:161-74.

Tresch DD, Sims FH, Duthie EH, Goldstein MD, Lane PS. Clinical characteristics of patients in the persistent vegetative state. Archives of internal medicine. 1991;151:930-2.

Vakkuri A, Yli-Hankala A, Talja P, Mustola S, Tolvanen-Laakso H, Sampson T, et al. Time-frequency balanced spectral entropy as a measure of anesthetic drug effect in central nervous system during sevoflurane, propofol, and thiopental anesthesia. Acta Anaesthesiol Scand. 2004;48:145-53.

Vanhaudenhuyse A, Noirhomme Q, Tshibanda LJ, Bruno MA, Boveroux P, Schnakers C, et al. Default network connectivity reflects the level of consciousness in non-communicative brain-damaged patients. Brain. 2010;133:161-71.

Voss LJ, Ludbrook G, Grant C, Sleigh JW, Barnard JP. Cerebral cortical effects of desflurane in sheep: comparison with isoflurane, sevoflurane and enflurane. Acta Anaesthesiol Scand. 2006;50:313-9.

Wu DY, Cai G, Yuan Y, Liu L, Li GQ, Song WQ, et al. Application of nonlinear dynamics analysis in assessing unconsciousness: A preliminary study. Clin Neurophysiol. 2011a;122:490-8.

Wu DY, Cai G, Zorowitz RD, Yuan Y, Wang J, Song WQ. Measuring interconnection of the residual cortical functional islands in persistent vegetative state and minimal conscious state with EEG nonlinear analysis. Clin Neurophysiol. 2011b.

Young GB. The EEG in coma. J Clin Neurophysiol. 2000;17:473-85.

Young GB, McLachlan RS, Kreeft JH, Demelo JD. An electroencephalographic classification for coma. Can J Neurol Sci. 1997;24:320-5.

Young GB, Wang JT, Connolly JF. Prognostic determination in anoxic-ischemic and traumatic encephalopathies. J Clin Neurophysiol. 2004;21:379-90.

Zeman A. Consciousness. Brain. 2001;124:1263-89.

Zhang XS, Roy RJ, Jensen EW. EEG complexity as a measure of depth of anesthesia for patients. IEEE Trans Biomed Eng. 2001;48:1424-33.

Chapter 3

# The Skin Neural Interface

Pierre Rabischong

Additional information is available at the end of the chapter

http://dx.doi.org/10.5772/51601

## 1. Introduction

The skin is the *smart dress* of all the body and represents its external limit in relation with outside and inside. Due to its particular rich innervations, it plays a basic important role as *polymodal neural interface*. Its structure is made by *three layers*. First the *epidermis* is a pavement epithelium without vessels and in a permanent growth by its germinative stratum pushing new cells to the periphery where the contact with air is drying them generating the stratum corneum of dead cells. That is why only free nervous endings can penetrate the epidermis generating a particular subtle tactile sense. Second the *dermis* is very rich in collagen fibers, vessels, hair roots, sweat glands and sensorial receptors of different types. Third the *hypodermis* has many fat follicles enclosed within fibrous capsules. Below those layers is the gliding *sub-cutaneous tissue* with connective and elastic fibers. Therefore the skin is a *movable dress*, but with some *fixation zones* to the skeleton or to some fibro-tendinous plans like in the palm of the hand or the plantar sole of the foot in order to guarantee safe grasping and locomotion.

It is important to remember that the skin has the same embryologic origin than the nervous system explaining some common physiological and pathological aspects. In fact, the *neural plate* originating like the skin from the *ectoderm* will give later after the development of the neural folds the *neural tube* progressively closed and enlarged at its cephalic end producing the five cerebral vesicles preforming the encephalon. During this embryonic process, the *neural crests* are isolated along the dorso lateral part of the tube to give the *sensory ganglion cells, the sympathetic ganglions*, the chromaffin cells of the *adrenal medulla* of the *surrenal glands* and some *migrating cells* within the skin described as *Langerhans* or dendritic *Merkel* cells responsible for *acquired immunoprotection*.

Finally the *smart transducer skin dress* allows to define five different and complementary functional neural interfaces: exteroceptive, proprioceptive, interoceptive, homeostasic and regenerative.

## 2. Exteroceptive neural interface: the multimodal contact

### 2.1. Touch and palpation

The skin can receive tactile information from the environment with contact of different pressure mode going from the light skimming touch due to the free epidermic endings till the deep pressure on the subcutaneous organs. It can also use their sensorial detectors to make contact with objects and move a sensitive skin surface to detect and identify the physical qualities of any structure defining the haptic function possibly assimilated to a cutaneous eye. Pain and temperature sensing are referring to other structures.

**A. The encapsulated cutaneous mechano-receptors**

A great deal of work has been done to characterize the different types of sensory receptors using physiological experimental techniques like microneurography and microneurostimulation as well as histological studies with the precious help of the electronic microscope. That means that we have at the present time a precise set of data concerning morphology and function of those receptors, but still a lack of complete understanding of the integration within the central nervous system of all types of sensations. Two functional types have to be considered: slow adaptating (SA) activated during all the duration of the stimulus and fast adaptating (FA) answering at the initiation and at the end of the stimulus. The richness of the skin sensitive matrix is also linked to the topographic repartition of the receptors in superficial and deep parts.

**A.1. The epithelial Merckel discs: (SA I)**

They are the smallest in the order of 2μm and placed parallel to the surface in the stratum germinativum or close to a hair follicle. The cell contains osmiophilic grains in relation with a neurosecretion and its surface is attached to keratinocytes by desmosomic links. They could be grouped in corpuscles or in Pinkus complexes and a single neurite can transfer information of few corpuscles. They do not have rest discharge and can give indication about the direction of the mechanical stimulus. It is important to make distinction between this mechanoreceptor and the dendritic cell also called Merckel and responsible for acquired immunoprotection.

**A.2. The Meissner corpuscles: (FA I)**

With an ovoid shape and a long vertical axis of 150μm, they are made by a superposition of Schwann cells between which are passing afferent interlaced fibers. Located mainly within the pulp of fingers, palm and plantar sole, they are sensitive to the direction, intensity and velocity of the mechanical impulses.

**A.3. The lamellous Pacini corpuscles: (FA II)**

They are the largest receptors in ant eggs shape of 2 to 3mm diameter and in fact visible with the naked eye. They are located in dermis and hypodermis of hand palm and plantar sole as well as in abdominal cavity and external wall of some big arteries and we will discuss later about their important functionnal role as pressure transducer. At the central part of the fifteen to thirty connective lamellas creating the classical aspect in onion bulb is a neurite with a neural plate. In addition some microarterial capillaries circulating between the lamellas are responsible for the renitency of the receptor and therefore for its sensibility. That can explain the balance perturbations in diabetic patient suffering of diverse microangiopathy changing the Pacini threshold.

### A.3.1. The automatic regulation of the grasping force:

That is an interesting neurophysiological aspect of the automatic control of motor functions related to the existence of a concentration of Pacinian corpuscles in the palm and palmar aspects of fingers. We studied this phenomenon in our biomechanical research unit using a cylinder test equipped with strain gauges in order to measure the grasping force as well as the acceleration. When a person is grasping by placing its palm around this unknown object and of course with unknown weight, the grasping force is generally higher than the minimum required. A second grasp of the same object shows a regulation with adaptation of the grasping force. If we increase progressively the weight of the object during the grasping phase by filling it with lead powder the force is normally increasing in relation with the variation of the weight. But we made this test in different categories of subjects and observed two extreme functional profiles: those who increase the force with a curve parallel to weight variation and those who have no regulation at all with a great initial level of force without change in relation with the weight variation. We also asked to the subject to voluntarily decrease the grasping force until the sliding of the object and we saw that a certain but variable safety margin exists to guaranty a safe grasp. That allowed us to identify the great differences between individuals regarding the precision and quality of regulation of this grasping automatic control. We established also a link with the important variations of the number of nervous fibers within the peripheral nerves and particularly in the upper limb and the hand. The mean number calculated on the counting fibers on cross sections of the nerves using a silver impregnation to visualize the myelin sheath in the different parts of the brachial plexus on 20 different cadavers was of 110000 fibers, but the individual variation on our sample was going to double or triple. The conclusion was that it is no equality among people regarding the quantitative aspect of the neural equipment not only in the peripheral nervous system but also in the central nervous system. That can also explain partially the inequality of mental aptitudes among individuals.

### A.3.2. The plantar force plate and the body balance regulation:

That is another interesting example of the mandatory automatic control of balance in vertical posture in relation also with the Pacinian corpuscles. Therefore man is the pilot of a very complex machine and in most of the case he is almost completely ignorant about its own anatomy and neurophysiology. Moreover the one who knows anatomy and neurophysiology is not functioning better that the ignorant pilot. That means that everything is made in the human construction plan to simplify at the maximum the conscious decision and command of action and to made unconscious the very complex technical problems to solve for the execution of motor tasks. The vertical posture on two feet (bipodal) or one foot (monopodal) is a good example of this full automation of a complex motor function. What we have to call the *postural servomechanism* has inputs and outputs.

The three inputs: visual, cutaneous and vestibular are redundants:

- the *visual input* takes unconsciously a vertical or horizontal reference line in the space and can alone achieve a stable balance. We demonstrated in our center that putting a person in a room without linear references create some specific optical vertigo, that it is also possible to reproduce by projecting in a dark room an inclinated line taking as a false reference by the person and generating a particular sensation due to the discordant perception of visual and cutaneous inputs.
- the *cutaneus input* is made by a string of corpuscles of Pacini located in the deep part of the plantar sole all along the ground contact part of the skin. They can detect the disequilibrium of the vertical posture on the two axis antero-posterior and lateral. This input is also able alone to assure a correct balance. Normally closing eyes in vertical position do not perturb the balance which is the case of blind persons. But in certain neurologic disorders like tabès characterized by a lesion of the posterior funiculus of spinal cord conveying the information of Pacini corpuscles, the equilibrium is impossible without the vision. This clinical test was described by Romberg.
- the third input is *vestibular* with the activation of the two accelerometers: angular with the three semicircular canals oriented along three orthogonal planes and linear with the utricular macula which is a gravity transducer allowing to maintain the head in horizontal position and the sacular macula for transversal movements of the head. The vestibular system is a complex accelerometer using a liquid technology with two liquids: perilymphatic and endolymphatic which also exists in the cochlea responsible as frequency analyzer for hearing, a completely different function, but with a common technical problem of precise osmotic regulation of those liquids. That can explain why vestibule and cochlea are linked in the same anatomical structure, the ear. Therefore the vestibule has a threshold as well as an inertia responsible for a remanence after stopping a movement. Only the vision can stop the vestibular activation avoiding a vertigo by resetting the transducer. In fact the vestibule in vertical posture can generate large oscillations for corrections in case of movements beyond its threshold. But its major role is to give a 3D trajectory for walking or running without vision.

The outputs are automatic muscular contractions by impulsions for correction of the disequilibrium in two directions. An EMG recording of anterior and posterior muscles of the leg and simultaneous recording of the center of pressure on a force plate can show clearly the proportionality of the muscular contraction with the importance of the disequilibrium in the limit of the 7° of acceptable oscillations of the whole body. These investigations are commonly done by the medical and non medical practitioners in posturology. An important literature can be seen on this modern topic.

**A.4. The Ruffini corpuscles: (SA II)**

They are *mechanical traction transducers* due to their elongated structure of 2 mm long with inside collagen fibers included in a liquid, surrounding a nucleus and with a thin capsule open at the two extremities. That allows some collagen fibers to go out and to be anchored and integrated within the chorion, making the corpuscles very sensitive to the mechanical deformation of the skin. A nervous fiber is penetrating within the corpuscle at its middle part and distribute fine ramifications inside. The neural reception field is large. This structure is very similar to this of the neurotendinous Golgi organ and play a great role in the body position and movement sense that we will talk about later.

A neurophysiological problem which did not find until now its solution can be called: sensorial convergence. In fact they are more receptors than afferent fibers to convey the information to the centers. For example looking at the finger innervations shows a great quantity of mechanoreceptors and largely less sensitive fibers within the two median and ulnar nerves. We have seen that several Merckel discs can corresponds to only one neurite, but for the other corpuscles the ratio 1/1 is the rule. The point is to know if different corpuscles types can be linked on the same fiber or if different topographical levels of same receptors can be associated. Presumably the answer has to be found in the organization of the somatotopy of thalamus and cortex identifying the different neuronal fields and their functional specificity. Anyway the Weber test exploring the identification of two separate contact points is in direct relation with this problem because the perception of a double contact is directly linked with the stimulation of two different neuronal fields. In addition a normal overlapping of perception fields exists and it is needed to get a complete anesthesia of a skin territory to cut three successive sensitive roots corresponding to three dermatomas.

**B. The temperature and pain receptors:**

Even if the two systems are specific, they are closely linked within the central nervous system. The temperature sensing is in relation with free endings with dilated end in cone or bulb shape in epidermis and mainly dermis. They are originating from Aδ myelinated fibers of small caliber of 5μm for cold and C amyelinic fibers of 1,5 μm for warm.

Regarding pain, the technical problem seems to be more complicated. Pain has to be considered basically first of all as a *protection system* generating a priority signal travelling as fast as possible within the nervous system in order to induce withdrawal reflexes or shunning reactions. This important *alarm system,* existing in all animals, requires a precise location of the injured part of the body to adjust the protective answer in the best possible conditions. That means a mandatory projection on the area 3 of the somato-sensory parietal cortex. On the other hand, specific nociceptors made by Aδ and C fibers were identified with slow conduction.

Therefore the question is to know if a supraliminal stimulation of a mechanoreceptor can generate a pain signal or if it is needed to think that a normal field reception is doubled by a nociceptive field ? presumably the truth is between. For example pinching the skin create a specific sensation which become painful if the pinching forces are stronger or putting a hand under water allows to identify the temperature of the water which can also become painful if increasing too much. That anyway allows to understand why temperature and pain are linked in the same central pathway and also the existence within the dorsal horn of the spinal cord of two types of nociceptive neurons. The first category is the specific nociceptive neurons which are located only in the layer I and have a little receptive field without overlapping. The second is the convergent neurons or also called WDR cells (wide dynamic range) or trigger cells or multireceptive neurons which are mainly within the layer V, have a large overlapping receptive field and are able to generate sensitive summation phenomenon explaining some projected pain like in arm in case of angor or in testicle in case of nephritic colic. Those convergent neurons have also a peripheral zone able to generate inhibition by non nocive stimulation. In addition to the neuronal activity, it is important to mention a very rich neurosecretion like excitatory aminoacids (glutamate or aspartate) or inhibitory like GABA or neuropeptides like substance P, enkephalin, somatostatine ...

## 2.2. The central neural pathways

Two different systems are corresponding to the two different aspect of tactile sensation.

The first is called *epicritic sensibility* and characterize a *precise body localization* and functional identification in relation with *touch contact discrimination, goniometric* and *statokinetic sense*. The signals are travelling within the dorsal column of the spinal cord along the *medial gracile fasciculus* for lower limb and abdomen and *lateral cuneate fasciculus* for upper limb and thorax to reach the two corresponding nuclei in the medulla. Then the fibers after synapses are crossing the mid line to create the *medial lemniscus* going to the *thalamic ventral posterolateral nucleus* in its pars oralis (VPLo). From the thalamus which is the convergent system of all the sensibilities except the olfaction, the fibers are projected on to the primary somatosensory cortex located on the parietal post central gyrus with the specific area 1 and 5 for the body scheme which is cutaneous and not muscular, area 3 for a precise body localization and area 2 for statokinetic perception (position and movement) including the segment goniometry. It is possible to find on the post central gyrus the same disproportional topographical representation identified by cortical electrostimulation on awake patients made by the Canadian neurosurgeon Penfield (motor and sensitive homunculus).

The second system is called *protopatic sensibility* and concerns *temperature, pain* and *crude touch* conveyed by Aδ fibers articulated in the posterior horn with lamina I and IV and V (nucleus proprius) and C fibers with lamina II and III of the substantia gelatinosa and VII and VIII. Then they travel within the dorsal and ventral *spinothalamic tract* (extralemniscal way) which is placed in the medulla and pons laterally to the medial lemniscus with whom its reach the thalamic ventral postero-lateral nucleus (VPL) in its pars caudalis for the ventral tract and in its pars posterior for the dorsal tract. In addition to the spinothalamic tract representing the alarm system mentioned before is the spinoreticulothalamic tract containing mainly C fibers which goes to the medullar, pontine and mesencephalic nuclei of the reticular formation (17 identified separate nuclei) and periaqueductal gray matter (rich neurosecretion within LCR). Finally this tract reach the reticular nuclei of the medial thalamus (intra and parafascicular) and then the anterior cingulate cortex (area 24) and close prefrontal cortex. That explains the two specific part of the pain sensations: first the *alarm system* well localized in the body with a discrimination of pain origin (stinging, cutting, burning ...) and second the *emotional component* possibly going to the *suffering* in case of chronic pain. Finally the central control of pain is made by three centers:

- the *spinal cord posterior horn* connected with the spinal ganglion which is the first pain processor unfortunately unknown by most of the spine surgeons operating on the vertebral disc. Some active inhibition process described by Melzack and Wall in 1965 as the *gate control theory* concerns the possible action of skin large fibers Aβ on the neurons of the substantia gelatinosa closing the door of the spinothalamic tract. That also can be done surgically as demonstrated by Marc Sindou.
- the *reticular formation of the brain stem* responsible for neurosecretion and activation/inhibition for ascending and descending pathways with three columns: *medial* with the 6 raphe nuclei with an important neurosecretion mainly serotonin, *central* with 5 nuclei in relation with motricity and *lateral* with 6 nuclei related to afferences. Even if we know precisely the morphology of those nuclei, more scientific investigations are needed to understand completely their specific functional activity.
- the *selective filter of the thalamus* in which 70% of the relay neurons of the VPL and VPM receive cutaneous inputs with roughly 20% of nociceptive specific neurons, 30% of low threshold mechanical SA and FA receptors and 50% of convergent WDR neurons in relation with non-noxious and noxious stimuli. The large diffusion to all the cortical areas of the pain signal is depending first to its localization by area 3 of the parietal post central gyrus.

## 3. The proprioceptive neural interface: The skin goniometer

As defined by Sherrington, the proprioception is the self sensibility of the body. In other words, the stimulus is not coming from outside but from inside of the body. That concerns essentially the perception of position and movement of all parts of the body. We have done in our research center many investigations on robotics and have had the privilege to cooperate with industry and particularly with the French Renault car factory which started its industrial robotic activity in 1974.

In order to better understand the technical problem in human, we will use a robotic model:

### 3.1. The robionic model

We created the term of Robionic in 1992 at the occasion of a robotic symposium in Singapore. That concerns the association of robotics, biology and electronics and was more appropriate than the term of bionics used in the sixties by the americans. At the present time, the engineers are talking about mechatronics. The name robot which means work was introduced by Karel Tchapek in 1922 in its theater performance called "the Universal Robots of Rossum". An industrial robot is a manipulator with several degrees of freedom (DOF). Some, considered as intelligent, are equipped with artificial sensorial systems, vision and tactile sensibility, allowing them to be adaptable to the unpredictable variations of a provided technical programme. The human limbs are also polyarticulated systems with many DOF and it is acceptable to stipulate that the control problems of human joints are of the same nature than the control of a robot, with of course some important differences regarding the type of actuators and the structure of the mandatory transducers. Two interesting transfers of knowledge can be taken in consideration:

**A. From living to artificial**

that is concern with the possible mimic of some living systems (biomimetism) like for example the compound eye of the fly which has 3200 optical microunits called ommatidies having a little lens as well as neural substrate with some specialized units in the detection of a particular direction of movement. The neural integration of the visual information is particularly complex but give to the fly a fantastic instrument to detect movement of objects or optimal trajectories for flying. Unfortunately a posterior dead angle of 7° make possible to catch it even if its reaction velocity is superior to man. A research team of Marseille was using this technology to design a special visual polydirectional transducer for mobile robot. Another example of biomimetism is the copy of articulated legs of animals to design legged machines including the present bipedal robots developed particularly in Japan for home services.

**B. From artificial to living**

this transfer is more interesting for us to understand the technical problems of human motor control. In fact to drive the terminal organ of a robot in a 3D space in order to grasp and manipulate objects, it is mandatory to find the correct algorithm of command and write the complex equations for that. Two basic information are needed: the state of the motors and the angulations of joints. In industry, the motors are commonly or electric or hydraulic. In both cases, they are reversible by inversing the electrical current or changing the hydraulic pressure. That means that the state of the motors can be identified by the measurement of the intensity of these two parameters. Regarding the angulations of the joints, it is easy to measure it by using linear or angular potentiometers placed on the axis of the joint and all possible forms and resolution commonly exist in the numerous catalog of components. It is now interesting to transfer these notions to the human manipulator control.

### 3.2. The human motor control

first of all, it is important to analyze the differences between the human manipulator and the industrial. It is also a polyarticulated structure, but in general with largely more DOF: 2 to 6 for a robot and until 31 for the human upper limb (9 for shoulder/arm/forearm/carp and 22 for hand). Concerning the actuators, muscles are viscoelastic, non reversible and non linear. That means that two actuators are needed for a single DOF: agonist and antagonist which is more complicated than the reversible industrial motors. They are roughly 600 muscles actuators in the body. The force is given by the shortening potential of the muscular fibers which cannot exceed one third of the length explaining the mode of construction of the different muscular plans which cannot be built using the best mechanical conditions. The viscoelastic structure of muscular fibers is made by the repetition of two components: a black disc made in contractile protein like actino-myosine able to reduce the length and a white disc made in elastin allowing a great flexibility and good absorption of mechanical stresses. For this reason the whole system is called striated muscle. It has the great advantage to be able to move without noise which is not the case for industrial motors.

The *motor command* is based on the concept of the *motor unit* representing the number of muscular fibers activated in on/off mode by a single motor neuron. Therefore the value of the different motor units is not uniform. In a muscle moving the eye ball they are 25 muscular fibers for a motor neuron and in the muscle on which we are sitting the great gluteus muscle around 6000 fibers for a motor neuron. That explain one of the basic rules of the organization: the *proportional control* by a variable *recruitment* of new motor units in relation with the type of motor task and the force requirement precisely controlled by the central nervous system and particularly by the cerebellum. In addition, the central nervous system has to know for an appropriate motor control the two pertinent information mentioned before for robot: the state of the motors and the angulations of joints:

**A. The state of the muscular actuators**

they are three possible states of muscles: relaxed, contracted, stretched. The sensitive parameter in this measurement is not the length as some physiologists still believe but the stiffness. This point is particularly important to be correctly understood. Therefore the optimal transducer is the *muscle spindle* made by few small striated fibers placed in a fibrous capsule attached to the muscle. Its length is in the order of 1 cm which make possible its microdissection under microscope. The intrafusal muscular fibers are innervated by gamma motoneurons entering at one of the extremity and giving the sensibility of the transducer. Sensitive neural fibers type Ia are fixed on the muscular fibers: at their equatorial part for the annulo-spiral fibers and middle part for the "en grappes" endings. Those nervous fibers are reaching the anterior horn of the spinal cord as fast as possible using a monosynaptic junction with the alpha motoneurons responsible for the contraction of the extrafusal muscular fibers of the muscle concerned. In fact when pulling a muscle with a traction on the muscle spindle, a muscular reflex contraction occurs which is called *myotatic reflex* (or stretch reflex of Sherrington). This basic reflex is not made only for exploring the motor control using a hammer with percussion on tendons like the neurologists are commonly doing, but it is the basis of the peripheral adjustment of the level of force needed to achieve a particular task. The decision of action initiated within the premotoric area of the brain is followed by the right choice of actuators made by a cortico-cerebellar loop, the right balance between agonist and antagonist controlled by the intermediate cerebellum and the correct level of force determined by the muscle spindles. The activity of the gamma motoneurons regulate the tension of the intrafusal muscular fibers explaining a possible hypertonia or hypotonia. In addition the inferior olive, a great nucleus of the medulla in pleated cortex shape, is playing the role of a corrector of errors in real time thanks to their connections with spinal cord and cerebellum.

All the muscles have muscle spindles except the vocal cord which is vibrating at high frequencies (20 to 20000 Hz) and is controlled by the hearing function and facial muscles responsible for mimics which are included within the facial skin and controlled by the trigeminal nerve in charge of the sensibility of the face. The ocular muscles and the lombrical muscles of the hand are very rich in those proprioceptors. Obviously in normal conditions, the myotatic reflexes are controlled by the central nervous system (spinal cord, brain stem and cerebellum). For example doing flexion of the forearm on the arm requires to inhibit the reflex on the triceps muscle (reciprocal innervations) allowing the biceps to move freely. That explain the *spasticity* which occurs in paralyzed patients by spinal cord injury, which made difficult the mobilization of the joints due to the lack of reciprocal inhibition of the myotatic reflex. In certain clinical cases the spasticity can be helpful like for standing up. But it can create, in the upper limb, spastic contractions in flexion with progressive fibrosis of the muscles.

**B. The angulations of the joints**

according to what we demonstrate before, the muscle spindles cannot measure the length of the muscles and even so, it doesn't exist within the brain a library of all the muscle skeletal insertions with the distance to the rotation axis of the joint allowing by a geometric calculation to know the joint angle value. In addition we commonly represent the muscle by a vector made by an arrow with a direction and an intensity which is a typical human language not understandable by the brain. The ligaments as well very rich in mechanoreceptors are not able to measure angle joints because they are not extensible and are redundant like in the carpal joint. They have to be considered as joint movement limit indicators, which explain painful sprain in case of over traction of the joint. The interesting solution is to use skin as a goniometer. In fact, they are many Ruffini transducers in the periarticular skin which have the same histological structure than the Golgi organ and are sensitive to the mechanical deformation of the skin of all the body segments in position and movement. The skin is movable thanks to the subcutaneous connective tissue but fortunately also fixed to skeleton and some tendinous sheaths like in the palm or plantar sole of the foot.

This important goniometric role of the skin can explain why the motor key board of the area 4 in the precentral gyrus is very close and linked with the sensitive key board of the areas 1,2,3,5 of the post central gyrus, generating a close loop control regulation that we called stato-kinetic loop. The same disproportional representation (homunculus) of muscles and skin territories exists in the two key boards, as demonstrated by Penfield after cortical electro-stimulations on awake patients. A great face corresponds to mimics and speech. A large hand with a great thumb is in relation with grasping function. A little lower limb representation is placed in the interhemispheric fissure presumably due to the automatic control prevalence of this limb, which also explain the relatively fast restoration of some form of walking in patients after stroke. The hemi-negligence syndrome, observed in hemiplegic patients, is in reality an alteration of the sensitive key board perturbing the position and movement sense. In normal conditions, this stato-kinetic loop allows precisely to know where we are and where we go at any time.

Some experimentations can also demonstrate the cutaneous goniometry by anaesthetizing periarticular skin territory. In this case, the person cannot precisely localize in 3D space without vision a segment of the body, like we observed for ankle joint and finger joint. On neurophysiological point of view, that reinforce the idea that muscles cannot give angulations' data, even if some physiologists reported projections of muscle spindles output on area 5 of the somato-sensory cortex.

They are also pathological arguments to validate that. The paraplegic patients with complete spinal cord functional section have no sensibility and they cannot perceive consciously the position and displacement of their lower limbs. That is called *asomatognosia* which can also be noted in tumors located in the parietal lobe. The patients are not paralyzed and can move freely upper limbs, but without vision they cannot identify position and movement of limbs. In addition, the post surgical scars particularly on knee, abdomen and back spine can disturb the skin goniometer and require some special resetting rehabilitation techniques in order to suppress pain or motor functional disorders sometime in the contra lateral side.

Finally, the *body scheme* that we have normally in our mind is not in relation with muscles but with skin and vision. As we mentioned before, muscles are consciously perceived only when they are painful in relation with C fibers between muscular fibers called metaboreceptors, corresponding to their sensibility to chemical factors like lactic acid accumulated after strong muscular exercise. We also command voluntarily and consciously movements and not muscles and we doesn't need to know we have muscles to achieve very complex tasks.

## 4. The interoceptive neural interface: The visceral mirror

The viscera placed within the thoraco-abdominal cavity are controlled by the vegetative nervous system with the two sympathetic and parasympathetic polarities on an unconscious automatic mode. Therefore their functional disorders can be expressed by clinical symptoms among which pain is the most frequent. But according to the poor conscious perception of viscera due in great part to the impossibility to feel or see them, the pain alarm of clinical disorders logically is projected on skin, which is on the contrary very precisely accessible for the people. Therefore it is classical to describe painful sensation in the right abdominal fossa in relation with appendicitis, right scapular pain with gall bladder problem, lumbar pain with nephritic colic, left abdominal fossa with sigmoiditis, left arm with coronary infarct... Anyway that not excludes real pain of internal organs like ureter, urethra, bronchus or Fallopian tube. But the close relationship between skin and viscera is a reality that Henri Jarricot (1971) was demonstrated by the technique of "palper-rouler" which is to pinch abdominal skin fold to detect a specific metameric pain corresponding to a particular viscera. He made a precise map allowing also by skin manipulation (reflex dermalgia) in the most painful area to get good clinical result. For example, making this manipulation on the area of gall bladder placed on the right part of the abdominal wall below the last ribs and using at the same time a stethoscope to listen the middle abdomen allows to perceive the contraction of the gall bladder and its expulsion in the duodenum with pain loss. The same maneuver can be done on the skin of left iliac fossa to treat the typical pain related with colo-sigmoid spasm. The modification in those areas of the tactile perception of the skin is related to oedematic infiltration by activation of sympathetic and C fibers which are connected with the vegetative visceral intermediate zone of the spinal cord. That is also important to know in order to avoid diagnostic mistakes.

## 5. The homeostasic skin: The neuro-vascular bundles

This functional aspect of the skin has some specificities which are not well known even if some recent scientific work has demonstrated the physical, histological and physiological reality of neuro-vascular bundles that Chinese called long time ago acupuncture points. This ancient technique is more and more used in medicine and a new scientific orientation of research allows to modify the Chinese tradition in order to make it more acceptable by modern medical community. Niboyet in 1963 demonstrated the less electrical resistance of the acupuncture points which was confirmed by a series of measurement made in direct and sinusoidal current by Terral in the Unit 103 of INSERM in Montpellier. The use of a curve plotter and of an exploratory electrode equipped with a force strain gauges bridge allows to record very precisely the relation between pressure on the skin and electrical equivalent circuit changes corresponding to low electrical resistance in the order of 10/560 kΩ. A first hypothesis to explain this phenomenon was to think about a skin surface effect related to a secretion of sweat glands as pointed out by some researchers. But the persistence of the current modification after cleaning the skin with ether/acetone and similar positive test on the skin of fresh cadavers obliged to predict a specific subcutaneous structure.

An *histological study* was performed by Terral and Auziech in 1975 in the faculty of medicine of Montpellier. Before operating on serial histological sections, the point electrically localized was injected with black ink in order to be sure of its precise localization. Then different staining methods were used (Coujard-Champy and silver impregnation) allowing to identify what were called "neurovascular bundles" (NVB) with, visible on serial sections:

- lax connective tissue with a shaft in the dermal layer
- different types of cell: fibrocytes, fibroblasts, mastocytes, histiocytes, Langerhans or Merckel cells, APUD cells
- intricate network of myelinated and unmyelinated nervous fibers among microblood vessels (arterioles, veins and lymphatics)
- radiating matrix into the epidermic basal layer indicating epidermic connections

This study was completed by an *electron microscope* investigation showing clear local endocrine and enzymatic activities particularly adrenaline secretion after electro-stimulation of the point. This original neuro-vascular interface was always found below the detected points with some variations particularly regarding those able to generate analgesia.

Finally after these physical and histological arguments, it is possible to accept the scientific demonstration of the real existence of the NVB (acupuncture point) even if the meridians, that the Chinese described with many details, doesn't exist anatomically. All attempts to use tracers like radioactive substances to prove their real existence were negative and finally they have to be considered as intellectual creations like the constellations in the sky which are lines joining stars or planets placed not on the same level and sometimes separated by light-years distance.

In order to get more arguments proving the possible functional action of NVB, a physiological experimental reproducible model was achieved using rabbit, which is an animal with symmetric locomotion of hind limbs. In fact generating a cutaneous pain signal on one side generates a double withdrawal reflex. That allows to have objective validation of a possible skin analgesia. After implantation of two needles within two NVB of a hind limb and electro-stimulation applied on the needles during twenty minutes, a real analgesia was observed. The animal is not paralyzed and can move on the ground. But the mechanical painful skin prick on the analgesic side doesn't create withdrawal reflexes, whereas on the other side a bilateral withdrawal was observed after painful stimulation. In addition, the delay between the beginning of stimulation and the analgesia strongly suggests a neurosecretion phenomenon. In order to validate this hypothesis, an injection of the serum obtained by blood centrifugation of an animal with analgesia was done to a naive animal. In a majority of the cases, it was possible to observe a real transfer of the skin analgesia almost in the same territory and a first biochemical screening indicated a possible role of an enkephalin. According to its regional action, it could be considered as a metameric antalgic neurotransmitter. Complementary investigations are in process to validate the result of this experimentation which can have interesting applications in the future for the regional treatment of pain disorders.

In addition, an *implantation of a microelectrode* after fixation of the rabbit head in a stereotactic frame was done within the parafascicular nucleus of the thalamus where the pain signals are projected. It was possible to demonstrate the suppression of the signals after stimulation of NVB and its persistence if the needles are placed few cm out of the points. This aspect obliged, for a good clinical efficiency of the acupuncture practice, to respect strictly this principle of action.

A problem remains which is to try to understand why such NVB exist in all vertebrates including men and what can be their functional role. Obviously it is not for a medical doctor to put a needle in and we formulated three hypothesis:

1. the *thermo regulation* is a complex but precise function which is very well controlled by reestablishing rapidly the normal body temperature for example after a muscular exercise. It is commonly accepted that an hypothalamic centre control thermo-genesis or thermolysis by reacting to the blood temperature feeding it. But it seems technically impossible to have only one thermostat for the thermoregulation of all the body

segments with some exposed parts to outside and others protected by dresses. That is why the NBV can play the role of peripheral thermostatic regulator able to modify the organ blood supply and particularly for the viscera which have as we saw a close functional connection with skin. Doing that they can modify the temperature in addition to the sweat glands secretion for thermolysis and the muscle shiver for thermo-genesis. Therefore modifying the blood supply of an organ means change its function and this process can explain a large part of the clinical efficiency of acupuncture on reversible functional disorders.

2. the NVB are located within the skin and it is normal to consider that they play an important role in the *maintenance* of it as neuro-vascular interface. As we will see later, the cell mobilization in relation with a cutaneous injury requires peripheral control units which can be those NVB. It was demonstrated as a clinical argument the efficiency of acupuncture needling around a bed sore to close the wound. In addition the connection between NVB and Merkel cells which are responsible for acquired immunity could be integrated in this skin maintenance.
3. even if the meridians have to be interpreted as virtual lines joining NVB, the unmyelinated fibers identified in are sympathetic fibers with predominant action on arterial diameter and in fact on blood flow as well as C fibers for pain transmission. The dermalgic reflexes of Jarricot described previously with their hyperalgic zones are clearly related to NVB. All the NVB are finally conveying different signals to spinal cord, reticular formation, thalamus and hypothalamus, representing a large network responsible for the management of what we call *homeostasy*. It can be defined as a state which is a maintained and regulated equilibrium of basic biological parameters controlled by the vegetative nervous system bipolar action and supervised by the hypothalamus closely connected with the hypophysis gland, representing the conductor of the endocrine orchestra. Therefore the functional entity of the whole body has to be understood as a very large, complex and intelligent neuro-vascular interacting system, fluctuating by time but conserving a form of homeostasic stability.

## 6. The regenerative skin: The healing process

That represents one of the most innovative biological auto protection of the body. Any form of rupture of the epidermic continuity generates a cascade of repairing coordinated events with a common finality to close the wound. The actors of this precise orchestration are local and migrating cells, growth factors and enzymes. The most frequent sequence of phases is as follows:

1. *hemostasis*: a tissue injury is commonly followed by bleeding. That induces the coagulation process with thrombocytes clumping, vasoconstriction in relation with vasoactive amines like histamine and serotonine, clotted blood after cleaving fibrinogen into fibrin and finally scab by dehydration.

2. *inflammation*: PMN (polymorphonuclear leukocytes) extruded from vessels are invading the wound in order to cleanse it and chemotactic agents are released like FGF (fibroblastic growth factor), TGF (transforming growth factor) and PDGF (platelet-derived growth factor). In addition, monocytes are exuding from vessels and become active macrophages which perform also this mandatory cleaning procedure using phagocytosis helped by their own secretion of TGF, cytokines, IL-1 (interleukin-1), TNF (tumor necrosis factor) and PDGF. This complex process of cell mobilization is going on few days and is characterized by some classical symptoms: rubor, tumor, dolor and calor. These symptoms are normally disappearing in few days if only the normal bacterial cutaneous environment is not modified by pathogenic germs introduced into the wound. But also in this case, the immunological defense can react positively or with a specific additional help by medical or surgical therapy.
3. *granulation:* four different and complementary events are occurring. First *fibroplasia* is the migration of fibroblasts into the wound in order to produce a new extracellular matrix necessary to support a cell ingrowth. Collagen fibrils are produced by a complex process starting by the precursor called tropocollagen cleaved by peptidases to give all form of collagen types I and III. Second the deposition of a *new provisional matrix* is performed and gradually replaced by a collagenous matrix, suffused with many fibroblastic components like fibronectin, hyaluronic acid, chondroitin sulfate and proteoglycans. Third an *angiogenesis* is needed to create a *granulation tissue* and is induced by a great quantity of growth factors like vascular endothelial, transforming factor β, angiogenin, angiotropin... Plasmin and collagenase are digesting basement membranes allowing migration, mitosis and maturation of endothelial cells able to create new blood vessels. This new vasculature is also stimulated by hypoxia following the injury and elevated lactic acid. Four is a *re-epithelization* by migrating epidermal cells from periphery using cytoplasmic actin filaments and dissolution of intercellular desmosomes separating epidermal and dermal cells. In this complex cellular movement at the growth speed in the order of 0,2 mm/day, the expression capacity of integrin receptors of epidermal cell membrane is interacting with a large variety of extracellular matrix proteins allowing to dissect the wound by isolating eschar from viable tissue and to bridge it.
4. the ultimate phase which can take few weeks or more is the *remodeling*. The migrated epidermal cells reorganize their basement-membrane proteins restoring their normal phenotype and reestablishing dermis attachment. A specific wound contraction occurs in relation with a very sophisticated phenomenon well described by J.W Madden in 1973 who identified a particular fibroblast phenotype called myofibroblast. It is made by large bundles of actin microfilaments placed along the cytoplasmic part of the plasma membrane with cell to cell and cell to matrix linkages in relation with complex growth factor interaction. Therefore these myofibroblasts have some similarities with contractile smooth muscle cells.

Finally the ultimate scar resulting from the described repair sequence has no more than 75% of the tensile strength of the replaced skin. In addition this normal procedure can be altered by abnormal factors like excess of collagen production which can generate hypertrophic scars and keloids or infections by pathogenic germs. In fact normally the skin has a great quantity of commensal resident germs living in a good intelligence with their living environment. When a wound occurs, a normal proliferation of germs Gram+ appears which can be replaced by germs Gram- and faecal germs which are integrated within the bacteriocycle needed for the cleaning phase of the wound healing. But real pathogenic germs can invade the wound generating abscess or necrotic tissue requiring an appropriate treatment eventually but not always by antibiotics or surgical approach.

This incomplete but consistent description of this regenerative skin function can clearly demonstrate the unsuspected complicated but intelligent organization of the skin, which cannot be, without a great difficulty, explained by random processes.

All these skin neural interfaces have been described in their normal state, but like all the organs of the body the skin have some changes in relation with age. We call this progressive degradation of structures by time: *ANATOCHRONESIS*. Skin aging relates to genetic, hormonal, metabolic and environmental factors. The epidermic cells are permanently reproducing and some age related DNA deterioration can generate a replicative senescence by shortening of telomeres forming the caps at the end of DNA strands. The consequence is that the epidermis is becoming thinner and more vulnerable. Regarding hormonal influence, the sex hormones are decreasing with aging and particularly for women during menopause the estrogen binding to receptors in skin are modifying the thickness, wrinkling and moisture of the skin. As demonstrated scientifically, the velocity of blood flow in capillaries is significantly reduced. The metabolic factors are playing a great role as well. The free radicals which are highly volatile molecules are participating to the oxidative stress, breaking down collagen, damaging DNA, releasing abnormally cytokines and participating actively to allergic reactions. An elevated blood sugar can also increase cutaneous anatochronesis by the process called *glycation*, in which sugars attach themselves to the amino groups of tissue proteins and particularly collagen creating AGEs (advanced glycation end products) which are very destructive for collagen fibers, losing elasticity and becoming rigid. A *matrix degrading state* progressively appears due to collagen degrading enzymes called MMPs (metalloproteinase's). That gives the particular aspect of aging skin. Moreover the gravity force acts on round organs like breast and buttocks often out of the plastic surgery possibilities. Wrinkles and fine lines in face deforming eye lids and mouth lips is a real depression motivation for elderly but a spectacular financial success for cosmetic industry. More dangerous are the deep perturbations of capillary circulation which explain, as we saw before, some structural changes in Pacinian corpuscles of the plantar sole justifying the important balance disorders in diabetic patients. The Langerhans cells responsible in the skin for the acquired immune defense can also be altered increasing the sensibility to infections. Finally the most dangerous environmental factor is the sun exposure producing long wave UV-A (ultraviolet radiations) and mid wave UV-B inducing oxidative stress and hyper pigmentation by melanin production representing the photoaging. The so appreciated tanned skin which becomes a must for a part of our society is in reality a real skin damage that it is also possible to observe on rural workers not for the same reason. Even if the sun exposure can be benefit for the vitamin D synthesis the real difficulty to apply the right radiation dose will push to prefer oral daily well controlled ingestion. In addition, tobacco use is damaging seriously the skin creating the typical smokers skin. The final consequence of this inevitable anatochronesis is that aging is never a progress nor a good motive for happiness.

## 7. Conclusion

Even if for didactic reasons the five aspects of the skin neural interface were presented separately, it is important to consider that they are functioning all together with many complementary links. That gives to the organ skin a great importance in the whole system. In fact skin is the largest organ of the body which is more than a barrier with outside world having enough mechanical resistance to support heavy stress and constraint. But also it has a very rich nervous equipment able to answer properly to the mandatory communication with the external environment as well as internal complex biological machinery. Therefore all medical actions for diagnosis and treatment are always done through the skin which has also a real anatomical continuity with mucosa of digestive, respiratory and sexual tracts. The abundant literature on it is with the diversity of research programs in progress all along the world the best prove for its major interest.

## Author details

Pierre Rabischong
*Emeritus Professor and honorary Dean of the Faculty of Medicine,*
*Montpellier, France*

## 8. References

[1] Rabischong P, Peruchon E, Pech J. Is Man still the best robot?. 7th International Symposium on Industrial Robots, Tokyo. 1977; Proceedings 49-57.
[2] Melzack R, Wall PD. Pain mechanism: a new theory. Science. 1965; 150: 971-979
[3] Sindou M, Quoex C, Baleydier C. Fiber organization at the posterior spinal cord rootlet junction in man. J Comp Neurol. 1974; 20: 391-408.
[4] Duvernoy H. The human brain stem and cerebellum. Wien: Springer; 1995.
[5] Jarricot H, Wong M. De certaines relations viscerocutanées métamériques ou dermalgies reflexes en acupuncture. Méridiens. 1971; 16: 87-126.
[6] Terral C. Douleur et acupuncture: de la recherche à la clinique. Sauramps médical. 2009
[7] Niboyet JEH. Traité d'acupuncture. 3 vols. Moulins les Metz: Maisonneuve. 1970.

[8] Nogier P. Introduction pratique à l'auriculothérapie. Bruxelles: Satas; 1997.
[9] Romoli M. Auricular acupuncture diagnosis. Churchill Livingstone Elsevier. 2009.

Chapter 4

# Sleep Spindles – As a Biomarker of Brain Function and Plasticity

Yuko Urakami, Andreas A. Ioannides and George K. Kostopoulos

Additional information is available at the end of the chapter

http://dx.doi.org/10.5772/48427

## 1. Introduction

### 1.1. Overview of spindles as thalamocortical (TC) oscillations

Spindles appear in the EEG as sinusoidal waves with frequency in the range 11 to 16 Hz. Together with K-complexes they are the hallmarks of NREM sleep and their appearance is taken as evidence of the onset of light sleep. Their specific distribution and exact frequency, changes in early and late sleep during the night. Sleep spindles are also known as "sigma waves" a term initially recommended (1961) but later discouraged by the International Fenderation of Societies for Electroencephalography and Clinical Neurophysiology (IFSECN), and redefined as a "group of rhythmic waves characterized by progressively increasing, then gradually decreasing amplitude"[1].

Spindles are one of the basic TC EEG rhythms appearing in sleep, these include the slower rhythms in the 0.05–1 Hz (slow rhythm), the 1-4 Hz (delta rhythm), and the 8–12 Hz (alpha and mu rhythms) .On the other side of the spindle frequency range we encounter the higher rhythms in the 16 to 25 (beta band), the 26 to 90 Hz (gamma band), the 100-200Hz bursts (hippocampal ripples that are associated with spindles) and the 300–600 Hz (ultrahigh-frequency oscillations) [2]. Although spindles have been the most thoroughly studied of these rhythms, in experimental animals as well as humans, with electrophysiological, metabolic, brain imaging and pathology, molecular genetic and computational modeling methods, their nature is still elusive. Their role has been debated for a long time but it is now believed that their contribution includes sleep promotion and maintenance associated to sensory gating, motor representation development, and cognition and memory consolidation.

The existence of two types of spindles were first described by Gibbs and Gibbs (1964), which differed in frequency by approximately 2-Hz; fast spindles, with a frequency of 14-Hz in the centro-parietal region; and slow spindles with a frequency of around 12 Hz, which are more pronounced in frontal region [3]. Recent studies using simultaneous EEG and MEG recordings have clarified multiple simultaneously activating cortical sources of two types of spindles in the centro-parietal areas [4-6], involving motor and sensory-motor cortex.

In this chapter we will review the basic mechanisms of sleep spindles and consider their possible uses as biomarkers for the state of the brain, focusing specifically on recent work on changes in sleep spindle activity during recovery from stroke.

## 2. Neural mechanism of sleep spindles during NREM sleep

### 2.1. Neural mechanisms underlying spindle generation

The existing fragmented views of the spindles' underlying mechanisms constitute a formidable puzzle. The main questions addressed so far will be covered in the following subsections.

Spindles and the neuronal mechanisms underlying their generation have been extensively studied in experimental animals [2,7] It is important to distinguish the mechanisms underlying the spindle rhythm generation, those producing the electrical sources of spindles recorded on EEG/MEG and those responsible for triggering, spread, synchronization and stopping this rhythm.

The **spindle rhythm** is considered to be paced from thalamus since it disappears after destruction of thalamus and survives in decorticated animals and even in thalamic slices [8]. The spindle frequency is basically determined by an interplay between the mutually interconnected GABAergic inhibitory neurons of the reticular nucleus of thalamus (RT) and the TC neurons (Figure 1), their intrinsic properties and their influence by cortical as well as brainstem ascending inputs. RT neurons impose hyperpolarization on TC neurons. This activates a nonspecific cation current, Ih, which depolarizes TC neurons and thus leads to activation of low threshold Ca++ currents (LTC) and bursting. The latter feeds back excitation on RT neurons, thus closing the loop and preparing for the next cycle. Each TC bursting besides feedback to RT imposes on pyramidal neurons an EPSP, which underlies each EEG spindle wave. The degree/duration of IPSPs imposed by RT on TC determines the intra-spindle frequency, but corticothalamic inputs have a decisive role on this pacing mechanism. This mechanism explained the old observation of two modes of TC activity, a rhythmical bursting and a tonic activity, the former prevailing (in the form of spindles or delta EEG waves) during quiescent NREM sleep and the latter in wakefulness. A simple common path for initiating the bursting mode is the hyperpolarization of potentially bursting neurons, so that Ih would be de-inactivated. Brainstem, hypothalamic, basal forebrain and the quantitatively most prominent cortical afferents to nRT neurons gate through this hyperpolarization the involvement of TC neurons in this cyclical interaction with nRT. This leads to the swich of TC neurons from tonic to bursting mode. Since the bursting mode is incompatible with faithful relay of sensory information to the cortex, spindles assume a gating role of dynamic sensory deafferentation during sleep.

Regarding the **electrical generators** of spindles, depth EEG recordings in humans have demonstrated superficial as well as deeper frontal cortical sources as well as sources in ventrobasal thalamus, which are usually but not necessarily synchronous to those on scalp EEG [1]. Animal experiments using depth profiles and intracellular recordings in thalamus and cortex have demonstrated that individual EEG spindle waves are scalp reflections of currents generated in cortex by EPSPs of cortical neurons. The elementary dipoles are considered to be generated primarily on the long apical dendrites of single pyramidal neurons; their extracellular current return branch contributing to EEG. These EPSPs are usually subthreshold depolarizations of apical dendrites and so give rise to smooth surface negative waves (type I spindle waves resembling recruiting responses). Only a few of the TC EPSPs progress from apical dendritic depolarization to deep soma and basal dendritic depolarization leading to cell firing and are shown on EEG as negative –positive sharper spindle waves (type II resembling augmenting responses). A spindle is usually a mixture of these two types of spindle waves [9]. These elementary dipoles will generate EEG spindles to the degree that they occur synchronously in a large number of neurons and in accordance to the rules of volume conduction in brain.

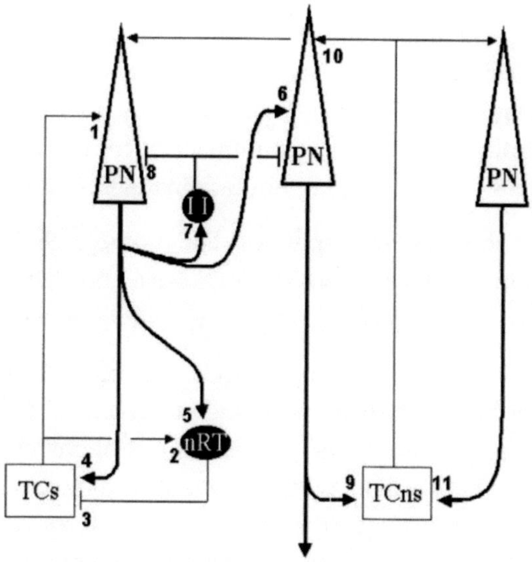


**Figure 1.** Main TC (TC) circuits relevant to spindles generation (simplified diagram based on Guillery et al., and Jones [10-11]). Excitatory connections are shown terminating with arrows and inhibitory connections are shown with bars. TCs and TCns are TC-specific and non-specific projections to pyramidal neurons (PN) in cortex. They are subject to feedback inhibition by nucleus reticularis (RT) and cortical inhibitory interneurons (II), respectively, shown as filled circles. TCs, considered as `core', 'first order' or `specific', excite PN of cortical layer 6 of the same TC sector (1) and RT neurons (2) and are inhibited by the latter (3). PN feed back to thalamus (4,5) and have a rich recurrent collateral network exciting other PN (6) as well as local inhibitory interneurons (7). TCns, considered as `matrix', `high order' or `non-specific', have similar connections with RT and PN of the same sector (not shown here), except for their rather non-discriminatory efferents to the upper cortical layers (10) rather than the fourth cortical layer. The PN of layer 5 (middle) constituting the main output of cortex can excite the latter type of TC neurons of remote sectors (9).

Several factors appear to **allow or instigate the appearance of spindles**. In the former one may include influences from brainstem, hypothalamic and basal forebrain to both TC and cortex, but the instigation role is attributed to cortical activation of RT neurons. This appears to occur in phase with a slow cortical oscillation (~0.75 Hz) [12] sporadically and during the A1 phase of the cyclic alternating pattern [13].

Cortical excitation of RT neurons is also found instrumental in the **spreading and synchronizing** spindles through TC and cortico-cortical excitation (Figure 1). It is noteworthy that the two function-related modes of firing characterize not only relay (specific) TC neurons but also the `non-specific' intralaminar nuclei. Cortical activation of the latter as well as of recurrent cortico-cortical excitation spread the spindle rhythm to wide cortical areas. The initially **waxing** amplitude of the EEG waves is grossly correlated to the amplitude of neuronal EPSPs and reflects gradual recruitment of more and more neurons in analogy to the augmenting and recruiting responses which are experimentally induced by activation of TC neurons in sensory-motor and intralaminar nuclei respectively, i.e. an initial specific activation of cortex leads to feedback excitation of nonspecific TC which will in turn project back to a much larger cortical area. This will then lead to the large amplitude EEG and hence the maximum amplitude in the middle of the spindle The **waning** is attributed to deterioration of synchronization of more and more extensive TC sectors, their asynchronous feedback to thalamus rendering RT neurons out of phase to each other, while also the recruitment eventually reaches a large enough number of cortical neurons whose feedback to the thalamus depolarizes TC neurons and thus terminates the rhythm.

Ascending arousal influences **disallow** spindles. For example cholinergic afferents from brainstem excite TC and inhibit RT neurons during awake and REM states, thus inhibiting the rhythm generation that prevails in NREM sleep i.e. spindles and deltas.

The **incidence** of spindles is reported to peak at a frequency of 0.2-0.3 Hz [14]. In longer time terms, spindles are under both circadian and homeostatic control [15]. Spindles density is decreased in early sleep stages (in inverse homeostatic relationship to slow waves). The same is observed after sleep deprivation, when there is also an increase in spindle amplitude and a reduction in intra-spindle frequency variability, which indicates a higher level of synchronization in TC cells under conditions of increased sleep pressure.

The incidence of spindles has considerable variance (1±40 s inter-spindle intervals in humans). Also variable is their topographic prevalence in the brain, their time of appearance in sleep stages, their association to other EEG landmarks (like K-complexes) and their dependence on drugs. All these suggest that spindles do not constitute a unique and/or uniform phenomenon.

## 2.2. Association/dissociation of spindles with other EEG waves of NREM sleep

The association of spindles the slow cortical oscillation (~0.75 Hz) [12] is proposed to be causative in the sense that this oscillation which is supposedly generated within neocortical networks, synchronizes neuronal activity into generalized down-states (hyperpolarization) of global neuronal silence and subsequent up-states (depolarization) of increased wake-like neuronal firing. With the beginning of the latter cortico-thalamic volleys are proposed to drive the generation of spindle activity.

During the A1 phase of the cyclic alternating pattern [13] spindles gather together with K-complexes. It is interesting that spindles are associated to K-complexes but are mutually exclusive with delta. The latter may be explained by the afore mentioned involvement of voltage-gated channels Ih and LTC, since the membrane can be only at one voltage level at a time. During sleep spindles the membrane potentials of TC neurons are between –55 and –65 millivolts, whereas delta oscillations occur in the range –68 and –90 millivolts. The progressive hyperpolarization of TC neurons during the course of sleep may explain the prevalence of spindles in early stages and delta dominance in stage 4 sleep [16]. K-complexes (the descending phase of their prominent negative wave) are associated with a population burst discharge of cortical neurons, including layer 5 and 6 pyramidal cells projecting to the thalamus. Such a strong and synchronous input may discharge reticular cells directly or indirectly and thus could serve as the initiator of sleep spindles [2]). In a recent study the incidence of spindles immediately following K-complexes was between 65-70% [17]. However in this study neither the probability of appearance nor the power of spindles correlated to the amplitude or any other feature of the K-complexes that preceded them. When K-complexes appeared spontaneously after the start of a sporadic spindle, the spindles were invariably shut down for the duration of the K-complex, usually being replaced by a short lived oscillation in the high theta frequency band. Also the spindles appearing immediately after a K-complex had invariably faster spectral frequency than the sporadic spindles. Such findings suggest that the association of K-complexes with spindles is strong but may be due to a common trigger rather than a causative interaction.

### 2.3. Spectral spindles frequency. Whence the appearance of two spatiotemporally distinguished types of spindles?

The observations of Gibbs and Gibbs (1950) [3] that the frequency of frontally recorded spindles is slower (about 12 per second) than that of spindles above the centroparietal cortex (about 14 per second), later confirmed in animals, suggest that several seeds of synchrony can emerge within the thalamus that are temporally coordinated by their corresponding neocortical networks. The different spectra of the two types are proposed to depend on anatomical differences (different thalamic rhythm generators and different distance from the cortical electrical generators). A possible explanation has been based on the fact that TC neurons in anteroventral and anteromedial nuclei, which connect limbic structures with cingulate and prefrontal areas, do not receive inhibition from RT but from zona incerta and other areas and so do not fire in coherence to other TC neurons during spindles [18-19]. The two types of spindle activity show different maturational courses [20] suggesting some fundamental difference.

Observing the actual intervals between individual waves of fast and slow spindles peaks on EEG we do not see a continuous spectrum with two peaks but rather a step like transition between two stable spectral frequencies even in cases the two types follow each other. More generally EEG spindles have been shown to display high intra- and inter-night robustness and stability of spectral frequency in individual subjects in spite of larger differences between subjects. This unique profile of spindles was suggested to be one of the most heritable human traits (heritability of 96%, not influenced by sleep need and intensity). Consistent with this suggestion is the demonstration that several diseases with strong genetic background are associated with changes in spindles, like Asperger syndrome, developmental dyslexia, Williams syndrome or malformations of cortical development ([21] and references therein). So, EEG studies propose for each of the two types of spindles a stable spectral frequency determined probably by the degree of hyperpolarization of TC neurons; determined in turn by intrinsic properties of these neurons. The latter as well as neuroanatomical differences are hypothesized to reflect genetically determined traits rather than sleep-dependent mechanisms. However the thalamic neurons membrane properties contributing to spindles rhythm display diurnal variation when recorded in vitro (more depolarization, bursting, LTC and Ih when recorded at night compared to the day [22]).

## 3. Electroencephalographic (EEG) and magneto encephalographic (MEG) findings, and other neurodiagnostic method of spindles

Sleep research is enjoying its second renaissance. Just like the first renascence in the late 50s and 60s the new one is driven by advances in accessing directly the correlates of electrical activity in the brain. The first renascence of sleep research was founded on the new capability of using EEG to extract a direct correlate of mass electrical activity of the sleeping brain. The pioneers sensed that something new was in the air with the advent of the new neuroimaging methods of PET and fMRI and remarkable progress in electrophysiology (EEG and MEG). This sentiment of great expectations is nicely captured in Jouvet's words: ".. so the majority of researchers are waiting with bated breath for the results of studies combining PET scanning, "functional' magnetic resonance imaging (fMRI), magnetoencephalography and tomographic electroencephalography …" [23].

We are now living this much awaited new era of sleep research, its second renaissance with the spotlight falling to the study of spindles for the reasons already outlined in the earlier sections. To appreciate the results obtained so far and even more importantly to sense the promise of things yet to come, it is important to understand what the new techniques can deliver and what they cannot and contrast this with what has been done so far. We will therefore describe snippets of new research obtained from different methods and point out in each case how these results add to earlier studies thanks to the new capabilities, but also how they are constrained by the limitations of the method. We will group the results in terms of the major categories of measurements in roughly the chronological order that each became available.

### 3.1. Non-invasive mass early mass-electrophysiology

The foundation of the modern neuroscientific study of sleep was laid by the questions posed by Henri Pieron [24] and Nathaniel Kleitman [25] about the physiological basis of sleep and the nature of regulation of sleep and wakefulness and of circadian rhythms. It took many decades though and critically the improvement in electrophysiological measurements that allowed the critical categories of sleep stages and sleep processes to be documented in an objective way. The key finding was of course the discovery of rapid eye movement (REM) sleep and its reproducible identification in any well designed study with polysomnography [26]. The cascade of discoveries that followed by the same pioneers together with William C. Dement, Michel Jouvet and many others continues for over a decade but by the 70's the field appeared to be running out of steam. In retrospect the big picture is easier to see and it can be summarized as the inability to connect the view of electrical events revealed by non-invasive mass electrophysiology mostly in humans and the detailed description of sleep control provided by highly invasive animal electrophysiology.

The source electrical activity is greatly distorted as it crosses the highly resistive skull, and as a result the EEG signal generated lacks spatial specificity. The EEG record at any one electrode is a crude average of real electrical events; at any one instance the signal could be due to any one or more generators spread over wide range of brain areas. The reader of sleep literature is used to EEG records that appear smooth with regular oscillatory patterns that cover wide parts of the scalp. This smoothness of the EEG signal is often interpreted as a consequence of uniformity in activity of the sleeping brain. In reality much of this apparent smoothness is a byproduct of EEG technical limitation and the efforts to limit them (e.g. through filtering).

A fine spatial and temporal detail in the pattern of activations would be smoothed by the passage through the highly resistive skull and in any case it would not survive the pre-processing of the signal. The absence of high spatial and temporal variability should not therefore be interpreted as evidence of absence. Spatial uniformity was however exactly what was implicit in the descriptions of brain activity within each of the major subdivision of sleep. This interpretation was of course at odds with the identification of fine spatial differentiation of mutually interacting nuclei at the brainstem and hypothalamus revealed by exquisite animal experiments of the pioneers. The reality of invasive neurophysiology was not of course inconsistent with the signal recorded by EEG but the interpretation of the latter was.

As is often the case in science, the animal neurophysiologists and the EEG researchers continue developing their own studies and terminology and practically ignored the inconsistencies between the implicit frameworks each society of researchers constructed. The unrecognized impact of this impasse probably contributed to the relative stagnation of sleep research that followed in the seventies and eighties as new methods were needed to bridge the results produced by the refined electrophysiology of animal sleep research and the gross electrophysiology of human sleep EEG.

In the early 1970s and through the 1980's mass electrophysiology was changing in fundamentals ways. First the advent of superconductivity and other technological innovations allowed measurements of the magnetic field generated by the human brain [27]. Magnetoencephalography (MEG) had some clear technical advantages over EEG, but the inertia of sticking largely to analysis techniques developed for EEG and the heavy pre-processing of the very noisy and limited data that early MEG hardware with only one or very few MEG sensors meant that the new capabilities were not exploited for almost a decade [28]. The advances in MEG, especially in terms of localization of cortical activity at the peaks of evoked response, spur a revitalization of EEG technology. In terms of instrumentation it eventually lead to computerized (paperless) EEG; which allowed long term recordings; in terms of analysis it lead to attempts to extract spatial information about the brain generators – it was not adequate anymore to describe the topology of the EEG signal on the scalp.

These advances augmented the effectiveness of standardization of sleep recording protocols. A proper sleep study had to provide enough electrophysiological records to produce a hypnogram, i.e. to divide a night's sleep into stages according to well-defined standards [29]. This classification essentially used the dominant frequency components and the big graphoelements to define each sleep stage. Sleep spindle activity is the highest during NREM 2 sleep stage and together with the K-complex are the two defining graphoelement for this sleep stage.

The contribution of MEG to the study of spindles has been limited in the 70s and 80s, partly because sleep studies with MEG are difficult and partly because partly because there is no timelocking mechanism for averaging and partly because there is little one can do that cannot be done with EEG with instruments offering limited coverage of the head with one or at most few sensors. Inability to identify spindles using a particular instrument and protocol was sometimes interpreted as inability to detect spindles with MEG [30] and different models were proposed to explain the apparent discrepancy between EEG and MEG spindle detection [31]. Eventually researchers recognized that when only few sensors were available the placement of the sensors is a critical determinant whether or not correlates of focal events in the brain will be captured in the measurements [32].

The advent of multichannel arrays covering a wider area, and especially the ones using planar gradiometer meant that events from at least part of the brain could be identified from the area below the sensor array. Indeed for the first time a concordance was reported for gross signal properties using such 24-channel array of MEG sensors and the EEG for simultaneous recordings from the scalp midline. However using the current dipole model for the generators no focal generators could be identified for spindles and slow waves [33]. The use of multichannel MEG hardware covering the entire head demonstrated that spindles involved activation of wide areas of the cortex. However, with modelling restricted to equivalent current dipoles all that could be done was to compare the relative occurrence of spindle-like activity in different parts of the cortex [34-36].

The EEG and MEG studies until the first few years of the new millennium have provided valuable information about the distribution of spindles in early and late sleep and the relation between spindle frequency and the phase of the slow cortical oscillations as described in section 2. In particular regularities in topography and timing were described in more detail than the original description of Gibbs, as already described in the previous section.

Defining cortical sources of spindles using simultaneous EEG and MEG recordings can provide valuable information on the role of the cortex and the underling neural basis and mechanism of generation of spindles [37] (Figure 2). Cortical activation centered in four areas, the precentral and postcentral areas in frontal motor cortex and parietal cortex of each hemisphere. Fast spindles were associated with more frequent activation of postcentral areas with stronger activation strengths, whereas slow spindles were associated with more frequent activation of precentral areas with stronger activation strengths. The differences in cortical activation patterns and activation strengths between the two types of spindles suggest that two distinct forms of spindle bursts propagate to cortex through different underlying neuronal circuits.

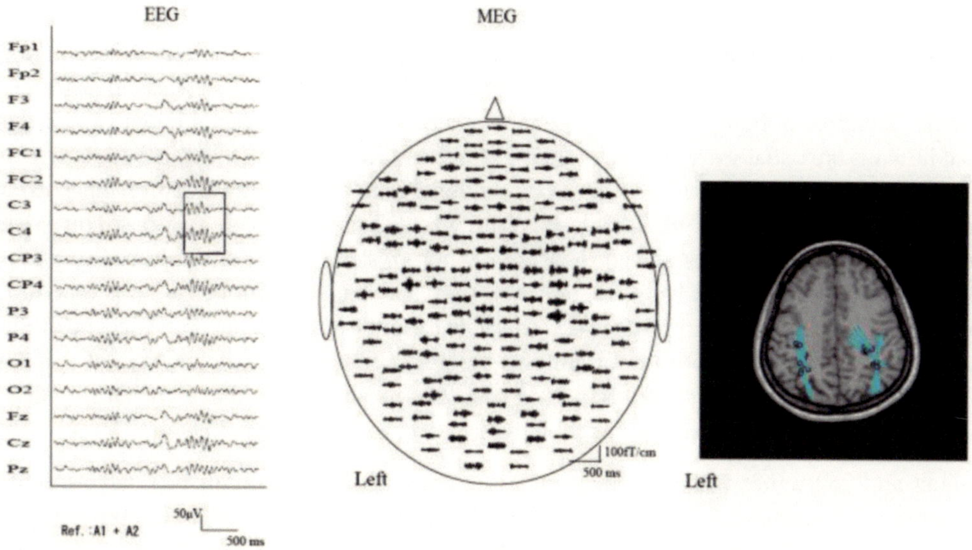


**Figure 2.** Symmetric distribution of 14-Hz fast spindles recorded with simultaneous electroencephalogram(EEG) and magnetoencephalogram (MEG). EEG shows spindles with a frequency of 14 Hz and amplitude of 30μV in the centro-parietal areas with the highest amplitudes in the central midline(Cz) and parietal midline(Pz) (Left) . Simultaneous MEG shows spindles with a frequency of 14 Hz and amplitude of 100.0 fT/cm distributed symmetrically in the MEG middle channels. The head is viewed from above (middle). The cortical sources of the same spindle were estimated as ECDs (equivalent current dipoles) with MEG clustered around the central sulcus of both hemispheres (right). Four locations consisting of the precentral and postcentral areas, in precentral areas of the posterior part of frontal cortex of each hemisphere and the postcentral areas of the parietal cortex activated. These cortical sources constituted the cortical distribution of spindles.

### 3.2. Hemodynamic studies (including combined EEG/fMRI)

PET does not have sufficient temporal resolution to probe in detail the evolution of activity correlated with large sleep graphoelements, so early studies have mostly focused on changes between sleep stages and awake state [38] with some attempts to characterize activity in spindles [39]. Advances in PET and particularly the simultaneous recording of the EEG allowed changes in PET signal to be correlated with changes in spindle activity, showing mostly CBF decrease in the human thalamus during stage 2 and SWS sleep, in proportion to the power density in the spindle-related sigma frequency range. A more recent study provided evidence for positive correlations in the thalamus and right hippocampus with sleep spindle activity [40]. Despite heroic efforts by PET researchers and some useful information obtained, it is difficult to draw firm conclusions about spindles from the PET data because the duration of the unit of measurements in PET is so much longer than the duration of spindles (< second) and even the periods of high and slow spindle activity (few seconds).

The advent of fMRI and its rapid development has revolutionized neuroscience and it has produced images of the sleeping brain that surpass even the most optimistic expectations of sleep researchers. The fMRI technology still relies on hemodynamic processes, but it has some clear advantages compared to PET. First, it allows much finer temporal and spatial resolution – its basic temporal unit is in the order of seconds rather than minutes; the spatial resolution is better and it can cover the entire brain, cerebellum and brainstem. It is also less invasive as it uses no radiation, although it still exposes the subjects to magnetic fields much higher than what humans are usually exposed to in their natural environment. Despite these advances, the use of fMRI in sleep research was limited for a long time because the rapid changes in the magnetic field create huge EEG artifacts. Without EEG it is difficult to do serious sleep research because sleep stages and the characterization of sleep events can only be done using EEG. This serious drawback has been removed with the development of methods that allow (nearly) simultaneous EEG and fMRI [41]. This new capability has lead to an avalanche of EEG gated fMRI sleep studies with important new insights about the nature and role of spindles coming with each new study. We focus on a couple of recent studies that arrive at significant conclusions and also point out the direction that research is following today.

Maquet and colleagues having done pioneering research on sleep with PET have recently moved to fMRI studies of sleep. The collaboration of Maquet's team with Schabus who has done some pioneering work on spindles with EEG has produced an excellent study where EEG gated fMRI allowed a detailed characterization of fast and slow spindles in terms of generators that are commonly active for both types of spindles and distinct neural networks that are activated for each one [42]. They reported an activation pattern common to both spindle types involving the thalami, paralimbic areas (anterior cingulated and insular cortices), and superior temporal gyri. No thalamic difference was detected in the direct comparison between slow and fast spindles but at a lower statistical threshold slow spindles showed increased activity in both thalami. Fast spindles showed thalamic activation in the common areas, but restricted to the lateral and posterior part of both thalami. At the cortical level identified significant common increases in activity were detected in paralimbic areas:

the left insula and the anterior cingulate cortex, bilateral superior temporal gyri (auditory cortex). The differences between slow and fast spindles were clear-cut. For slow spindles activity in the superior frontal gyrus was the only addition to the common activation pattern. The absence of additional frontal activity for slow spindles, what distinguishes slow from fast spindles with EEG, was attributed to a non-systematic participation to each slow spindle occurrence by any one frontal region. Fast spindles were correlated with activity in a number of areas in addition to the common activation pattern. These activations include areas around the sensorimotor strip, mid cingulated cortex and the SMA – all areas showing sensorimotor (μ) rhythm activity in relaxed wakefulness. Direct contrast between the two spindle types showed a larger recruitment of mesial-prefrontal and hippocampal areas during fast, relative to slow, spindles, a result consistent with the notion that fast but not slow spindles are related to learning (see below).

The complex relationship between spindles and specific activations was further explored in another recent study using EEG gated fMRI. In this study, 30 minutes of simultaneous whole brain fMRI data at 1.5 Tesla and polysomnographic EEG were collected while subjects were falling asleep in the MR scanner. From these data, 5 minute epochs were extracted each from a single sleep stage for more than 85% of the time. All in all, 93 epochs of a single sleep stage were extracted. 27 epochs during wakefulness, 24 during sleep stage 1, 24 during stage 2 and 18 in SWS were used for the final analysis. In addition to comparisons between stages and identification of regional changes of activity the researchers compared the connectivity network of timeseries extracted from timeseries of regional activations. Specifically the connectivity of the hippocampal formation with the rest of the brain was examined at different sleep stages and during spindles. The analysis failed to show increased hippocampal BOLD signal during fast spindles; instead, it was functional connectivity between the hippocampal formation and neocortical areas that increased during the appearance of fast spindles [43].

## 3.3. Invasive electrophysiology

Reviewing the development of our understanding of sleep spindles, it is becoming clear that important new insights were obtained when new tools became available that allowed a qualitatively new view of either local or global brain activity related to spindles or how local and global spindle-related brain activity relate to each other. While the foundations for the important developments in electrophysiology and neuroimaging were laid in late eighties, the mechanisms underlying sleep spindles (and TC rhythms in general) were seen in a new light thanks to pioneering work of Rodolpho Llinas and Mirca Steriade. Llinas and colleagues employed in vitro preparations to show that the membrane ionic channels endowed pacemaker properties to thalamic neurons. Steriade and colleagues employed in vivo experiments to demonstrate the importance of the nucleus reticularis thalami and its activation by the cortex in the generation and spread of the spindles rhythm, reviewed together in Steriade and Llinas [44]. This concept was refined as the "thalamic clock" theory [45]. The historical irony is that in spite of this revolutionary advance in understanding spindles made possible only by the synthesis of in vitro and in vivo studies, Steriade himself remained an outspoken critic of data collected in vitro [46].

Invasive electrophysiology in normal humans is of course not justified, but implantation of the brain for clinical reasons provides unique opportunities to access the brain directly. An important recent study has provided valuable insights by characterizing sleep spindles in humans by pooling together simultaneous recordings of intracranial depth EEG and unit spiking activities in multiple brain regions in the hippocampus and cortex of 13 individuals undergoing presurgical localization of pharmacologically resistant epilepsy [47-48]. The authors of these studies report that spindles occur across multiple neocortical regions, and less frequently also in the parahippocampal gyrus and hippocampus. Most spindles are spatially restricted to specific brain regions with topographically organized spindle frequency with a sharp transition around the supplementary motor area between fast (13–15 Hz) centroparietal spindles and slow (9 –12 Hz) frontal spindles occurring 200 ms later on average, consistent with earlier reports. They further report that fast spindles often occur with slow-wave up-states and that spindle variability across regions may reflect the underlying TC projections. They do not find a consistent modulation of neuronal firing rates during spindles [47]. They also report that most sleep slow waves and spindles are predominantly local inferring therefore that the underlying active and inactive neuronal states also occur locally [48].

### 3.4. Tomographic MEG and EEG studies

The results described above showed that spindle-related activity involves widespread activity in multiple cortical and subcortical areas. It involves characteristic times that are a fraction of the typical spindle period and the ones that characterize sleep periodicity as this is reflected in the sleep stages or the cyclic alternating pattern (CAP) [49] with characteristic phases of quiet activity and groupings of the large graphoelements that characterize each sleep stage. In short the study of spindles, like the study of much else about the brain, requires techniques that can look at the whole of the brain with time resolution from a few milliseconds to many minutes. The solutions described above were the ones that satisfied, at least partly, this need by combining more than one technique. As we will see below a more direct approach is provided by tomographic analysis of MEG and EEG data. The key transition came in the late 1980s and early 1990s for MEG with the introduction of truly tomographic analysis of multichannel MEG data [50] and a few years later for EEG [51]. Tomographic analysis of minimally pre-processed MEG data revealed a dynamic view of brain function [28, 52] that was very different to the smooth version of reality that was the consensus of decades of studies using equivalent current dipole analysis of highly pre-processed (filtered and averaged) MEG and EEG signals. The EEG and MEG community remained skeptical of tomographic analysis for a long time, despite convincing evidence converging from many directions: the agreement between results obtained with the analysis of the standard average and heavily filtered MEG signal with the results obtained after the same average and filtering operations were applied to the tomographic single trial solutions [52], the more consistent picture obtained with single trial analysis of MEG data with the variability encountered in animal invasive electrophysiology and the detailed justification of the methodology in terms of mathematical properties of the lead fields [53]

The change in heart came slowly and moved primarily by the demonstration of high variability with the advent of single-trial fMRI studies. Tomographic analysis of sleep data offers some great advantages, but the difficulty of sleep studies and the skepticism of the community posed great obstacles. The first such study with MEG focused on eye movements [54]. Attempts to characterize the graphoelements of NREM 2, K-complexes and spindles produced results showing activity in widespread areas as previously reported, but without much order to be useful for clarifying the role of different sleep stages. It was therefore decided instead to compare the quiet periods across different sleep stages with each other and with the state of wakefulness with eyes closed just before sleep [55]. These comparisons produced clear cut differences and notably a gradual increase in gamma band activity in the left dorso-medial prefrontal cortex from awake state through the four NREM sleep stages, culminating in the highest gamma band activity during REM sleep. It is tantalizing that this area or frontomedial areas close to it are implicated in memory consolidation in animals and in EEG-gated fMRI studies and shows increased connectivity with the hippocampal formation during fast spindles [43]. A meta-analysis of a group of 192 patients with focal brain lesions found the highest association between insomnia and left dorso-medialprefrontal damage [56]. Recent work from our team showed that this area is activated in the spindle range of frequencies during the core periods of NREM2 [57]. Specifically a direct comparison between activity during NREM 2 and awake state showed that the activity in posterior brain areas is substantially reduced compared to the awake state, while in the left dorso-medial prefrontal cortex – the centre of the area identified in the gamma band in the comparison between core states in REM and awake state – the activity is higher in the spindle range of frequencies (Figure 3A). A direct comparison between the activity during core states of NREM 2 and NREM1 showed increase in the spindle range of frequencies in the same left dorso-medial prefrontal cortex and in the thalamus (Figure 3B). The implication of this same area in the spindle range of frequencies during the quiet periods of NREM 2 stage provides yet another tantalizing clue hinting of some involvement of this area in the process of memory consolidation.

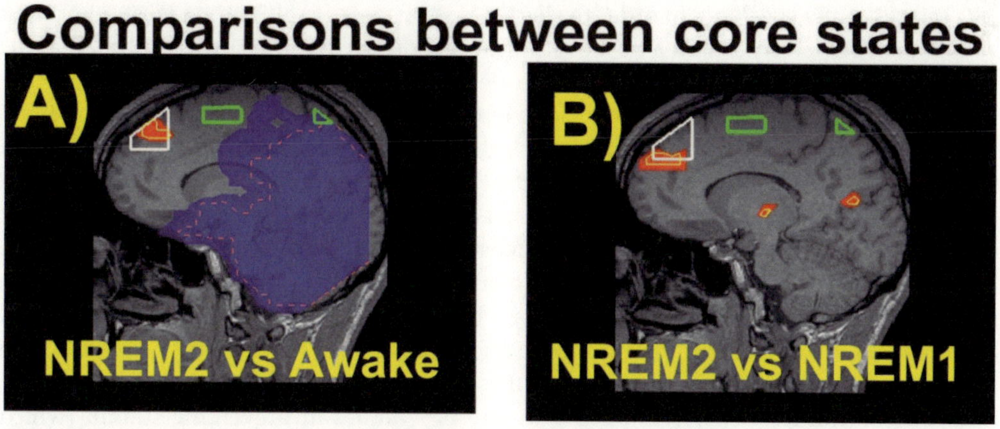


**Figure 3.** Comparisons between MEG recorded actications in the spindle frequency range (12-16 Hz) in core states of NREM2 and awake (A) and NREM1 (B) states. The thin yellow contour bounds the area that shows statistically significant increase in activity for all three subjects studied with $p < 0.0001$. In each case the areas identified in the comparison between REM and awake state in the gamma band are also shown by heavy outlines: the left dorso-medial prefrontal cortex (L-DPFC) in white and the pre SMA and precuneus in green.

The ability of EEG to be recorded simultaneously with fMRI and PET is an important advantage that has not yet been fully explored, at least not for sleep studies. It is nowadays possible to obtain some information about source generators from just the EEG signal [58-59]. Simultaneous EEG/MEG studies, notably from the team of Halgren and colleagues [60-62] are not only valuable in the richer information they capture, but they can also guide us how to reliably obtain information from more widely available EEG measurements, that are also more suitable for clinical applications as we will describe next. Finally, in closing this section it is worth noting that the increase sophistication in EEG measurements and experiment design are producing new information not just about the nature of sleep spindles but also about their role [63-64].

## 4. Stable sleep profiles in clinical and other conditions

### 4.1. Consciousness and spindles

As we gradually fall asleep spindles appear in the EEG at stage 2 NREM, when consciousness has evidently been lost. Their rate appears to correlate with the sleeper's tolerance to noise and sleep maintenance. The futility of correlating a physical to a psychological phenomenon withstanding, one may therefore ascribe to spindles a role of marker or neural correlate of the loss of consciousness. However, we are still searching for possible roles of spindles in the several and complex aspects of consciousness, its neurological levels, its variable memory contents and its physiologically or pathologically altered states.

Animal and human studies show that spindles are sleep maintaining events [65-66] that block the transfer of sensory information to the cerebral cortex during sleep [64], thus preventing sleep-interrupting arousals. The frequency of the spindles decreases with deepening of sleep and increases as sleep becomes lighter in each consecutive sleep cycle [68]. Teleologically speaking, in order to sleep, consciousness for all but the most relevant of stimuli must be prevented and a host of studies convince us that this is accomplished at the level of TC circuits [69]. TC neurons upon a decrease of ascending from brainstem mostly cholinergic afferents shift to a bursting mode of firing dictated by their hyperpolarization by RT inhibitory neurons the duration of which determines the frequency of their oscillation subsequently transmitted to and augmented by the cortex as spindles rhythm of 11-15 Hz (see 2.1.). While TC neurons are hyperpolarized and engaged in this bursting mode, sensory afferents are expectedly prevented from reaching the cortex, resulting in almost complete deafferentation, except for very strong or alarming stimuli [65]. In consistency to these observations, thalamic metabolic activity was shown to decline in association to increased spindle-frequency [70]. The recent observation (described in 2.2.) that spindles are invariably shut down for the duration of the K-complex and they appear right after at increased spectral frequency [71] support a role of spindles in preventing stimuli (which triggered the K-complex) to reach consciousness.

The definition of "Consciousness as information integrated" [72] leads to the question: Has our unconscious sleeping brain lost its dynamic complexity or its capacity to integrate the enormously diverse patterns of its activity into a unique consciously perceived whole?[73]. Among the arguments supporting the second of the two explanations is that spindles prevent integration of brain activity. Furthermore, their spatiotemporal dynamics and relationship to K-complexes as well as their involvement with hippocampus into a memory consolidating "dialogue" contribute to a very complex image of the sleeping brain [55]. During the whole of sleep, and especially in the second stage of NREM sleep, a dynamic confrontation of arousing and anti-arousing mechanisms is evident in the macro- and microstructure of the EEG. Loss and regaining of consciousness is continuously debated by hundreds of K-complexes and tens of microarousals each night, which are normally too short to fully awaken us, but constitute an opening of a dynamic window of information-processing, allowing some monitoring of possible threats. If the stimuli represent a lack of threat, sleep is maintained or protected partly with the help of spindles.

Anesthetics lead also to loss of consciousness - in the sense of turning the subjects oblivious to their environment - with different mechanisms depending on the drug used. One mechanism they partly share with natural sleep is apparently the production of spindles in a similar way, as several anesthetics hyperpolarize TC neurons (by activating 2PK channels and/or by potentiating GABA receptors) and halothane induced spindles are antagonized when carbachol is injected into the pontine reticular formation [74]. Spindling then causes a decorrelation between sensory input to TC neurons and these neurons' output to the cortex, thus contributing to the loss of consciousness.

## 4.2. Spindle-coma

Coma can be considered as a deregulation of the brain's arousal system caused by diffuse brain damage or by focal brainstem lesions. The arousal systems are 1) an upper level encompassing cerebral cortex and white matter 2) a middle level encompassing thalamus and upper brainstem and 3) a lower level encompassing lower midbrain and pons [75].

In coma the EEG shows a various patterns, a generalized slowing in the delta or theta range, alpha-coma, spindle-coma, burst-suppresion and epileptiform activity. In coma, regardless of pathology, a normal sleep-wake cycle is mostly disrupted or completely absent. However, the coma tracing may resemble normal wakefulness [76] or normal sleep [77]. The occurrence of spindles in comatose patients is refereed as spindle-coma is often caused by Central Nervous System (CNS) trauma, infection, and metabolic encephalopathy. The mechanism of abnormal spindling has been considered as midbrain involvement with sparing thalamic structures [77-79]. Silverman (1963) suggested that the spindle-coma in supratentorial lesions suggests relatively intact cortical function and a good prognosis [80].

Spindle-coma is considered as a benign form of coma, with EEG reactivity to stimuli heralding a favorable outcome. Spindles in comatose patients are best demonstrated during first few days [81] after trauma. They observed spindle activity in 91% of patients of post-traumatic coma, and 30% of these went to prolonged coma. Symmetrical occurrence of spindles was found to be of good prognosis, asymmetry and decrease of spindles showed a rather poor prognosis [81].

The presence of spindle activity after hypoxic or anoxic injury does not always indicate a good outcome. A more recent works supports these findings in comatose children and concludes that the reappearance of sleep patterns and sleep spindles is sign of good prognosis. In traumatic coma, these sleep elements are more frequently observed. Spindle coma represents a combination of physiological sleep and coma, the latter accounting for the failure of arousal. The neurophysiological mechanism of spindle coma is the preservation of pontine raphe nuclei and TC circuits subserving sleep spindle activity, with the impairment of ascending reticular activating pathways at the midbrain level that maintain wakefulness [82-84]. The presence of sleep-like patterns was shown to be indicative of a better outcome. NREM sleep elements, K-complexes and sleep spindles as well as rapid eye movements (REM) sleep elements alternating with NREM sleep elements were also indicators of a better outcome. Only monophasic EEG or a cyclic alternating pattern with absence of sleep elements indicates a poor outcome.

## 4.3. Spindles and epilepsy

Epilepsy and sleep disorders are considered by many to be common bedfellows. Sleep can affect seizure occurrence, threshold, and spread, while epilepsy can have a profound effect on the sleep/wake cycle and sleep architecture [85-87]. NREM sleep differentially activates interictal epileptiform discharges (IED) during slow wave (N3) sleep, while ictal seizure events occur more frequently during light NREM stages N1 and N2. Some types of seizures preferentially occur during NREM stage-2 sleep with spindles, and association between sleep and activation of epileptiform activity on EEG has been of interest to investigators for years. Medial temporal spindles are present in some children with focal epilepsy.and the frequency of spindles may be slower in patients with epilepsy, probably as an effect of antiepileptic drugs. Longer spindle duration has been observed just prior to seizures of nocturnal frontal lobe epilepsy. Overall IED rate may be increased during sleep with spindles, but the spatial distribution of spike frequency appears similar during wakefulness and sleep in children with intractable focal seizures. Thus sleep with spindles may decrease the threshold of emergence of IED activity diffusely rather than focally [88]. These EEG clinical observations are consistent with spindles representing a series of depolarizations of lower (type I) or higher (type II) firing capacity (riding on top of a DC negativity) and so constitute a state of relatively higher cortical excitability (see chapter 2.1.). The effect is rather non specific in the sense that the slow (<1 Hz) oscillation of NREM sleep, and in particular spindles, K-complexes and delta waves, share some features that may contribute to the aggravation of epileptic phenomena (see also clinical studies at the end of this chapter). These effects may be related to the dynamic bistability of neuronal membrane potentials and neuronal readiness for bursting and widespread synchronization [86].

Spike and wave discharges (SWDs), the electrographic hallmark of typical absence seizures, which are an integral component of several idiopathic generalized epilepsies [89], have been reported to occur preferentially during the light stages of NREM sleep, where the majority of sleep spindles are observed and in a reverse relationship to their rate throughout the night [90]. Gloor in 1978 [91] proposed that the same TC circuit producing sleep spindles would generate SWDs in states of cortical hyperexcitability [91]. The hypothesis was based in experiments in the animal model of feline generalized epilepsy with penicillin (FGPE) and developed further on the basis of in vitro and in vivo experiments, especially using rodent genetic models of absence seizures [92-95].

A more recent report [96] concludes that "the hypothesis that sleep spindles are transformed in SWDs now appears highly doubtful" based mainly on the arguments that (a) SWDs occur also during the day (during quiet awake state), (b) a compromised thalamic GABA receptors' function as a necessary condition for SWDs generation are not defensible and (c) spindles are initiated in thalamus while SWDs in the cortex. In our opinion SWDs do not develop from spindles (any more than humans developed from apes); they develop from the same TC circuit under different conditions - a thesis with solid experimental support to which the above paper subscribes to. The transition from spindles to SWD was just what was observed in the particular FGPE model (awake cats under fentanyl and curare successively injected with pentobarbital and penicillin [97]) and gave major support to the hypothesis that SWDs develop from the same TC circuits as spindles. Further more it was these experiments in FGPE, which first argued in favor of above (b - not compromised GABA inhibition) and (c - primacy of cortical mechanisms) [9, 69, 91, 92, 93, 99, 100]. One of the first robust observations, pivotal to the suggestion of this hypothesis, but not adequately followed up since, is that the spectral frequencies of spindles and SWD model co-varied in different cats displaying an impressively accurate for EEG almost 2:1 or 3:1 relationship [98] and most importantly that the transition from one to the other in FGPE was not continuous but step-like. This observation suggested that SWD may result from an increased cortical excitability which enhances the firing of pyramidal neurons to thalamic volleys of each spindle wave and thus activates recurrent cortical inhibition annulling the effect of the next one or two thalamic volley, i.e. it conferred to cortex the mechanism of SWD elaboration (as demonstrated and explained later in other animal models), through cortical recurrent GABAergic inhibition. This slower cortical rhythm was proposed to be transferred to the thalamus to gradually grow as a cortico-thalamo-cortical SWD rhythm. The experiments in the FGPE model that followed and supported this hypothesis have been reviewed [92-93, 100]. Further testing of this hypothesis was made possible when in vivo and in vitro studies revealed the exact mechanism of spindles generation in thalamus [44] (see chapter 2.1) and when this knowledge was applied to experiments on rodent genetic models of absence seizures [94-95].

In a general view, EEG alpha rhythm presents itself in awake state, when visual and other environmental stimuli cease; sleep spindles reflect the bursting mode of TC neurons which raise awakening threshold by blocking the weak sensory inputs, an effect further aggravated during delta waves in NREM N3; and finally SWD almost totally incapacitate awareness of and reaction to the environment either in awake or sleep condition and especially in the transition between the two. There is evidence suggesting that this may depend more on a top-down effect rather than merely being allowed by a decrease in arousal inputs from the brainstem [69,93]. There is little doubt however that all these rhythms - alpha, spindles, delta and SWD - (and not only) appear to cardinally involve cortico-thalamo-cortical circuits and bursting of TC and cortical neurons, albeit at distinct frequencies. The task is to understand why the frequency spectrum of TC rhythms is distinct rather than continuous and what is the role of internal (membrane and circuit) properties as well as external influences on this reentrant TC system in setting the frequency constrains, but also allowing, triggering, augmenting, spreading and stopping each of these rhythms.

The elegant experiments of Steriade and his colleagues identified the cortex as responsible for instigation, augmentation and generalization of spindles (ch. 2.1.) and this may be truer for SWDs [65], as explained above [9, 69, 91, 92, 93, 99, 100]. In spite of the long held view of a brain-wide synchronous start of SWDs out of a normal background, one of the most important recent discoveries in the field has been the identification of a cortical 'initiation site' of SWDs. A consistent cortical site of initiation of SWDs within the perioral region of the somatosensory cortex was demonstrated in rodent absence seizures. High density EEG as well as MEG and fMRI studies in patients with different types of idiopathic generalized epilepsy (IGE) has shown SWDs in discrete, mainly frontal and parietal cortical regions before they appear over the rest of the cortex [101-106]. These studies strongly suggest that the frontal lobe is important for the generation of the 3Hz corticothalamic oscillations Do spindles play a role in this new view of IGE?

In a study aiming to investigate the relationship between IED and phasic sleep phenomena in patients with juvenile myoclonic epilepsy, only 2.7% of IED emerged specifically through sleep spindles as opposed to 65% from K-complexes, while IEDs were both facilitated by increased vigilance (CAP - A phase) and promoted the appearance of such periods [107]. In a further study of childhood absence epilepsy [108] focal SWDs occurred mainly during non-CAP and CAP-B periods (periods of reduced vigilance) of NREM sleep, whereas generalized SWDs occurred during the CAP-A of NREM sleep and especially at the transition from reduced to enhanced vigilance of NREM sleep. Regarding the efforts to understand the relationship between spindles and epilepsy, these studies emphasize the importance of (a) mutual interaction between the two, (b) recognizing that different types of epilepsy may have different mechanisms and (c) the importance of observing the "bigger picture" in both time (i.e. CAP periods) and brain space, since both sleep and epilepsy by definition involve large brain circuits.

### 4.4. Spindles in dyslexia

Much of the interest in sleep spindles arises from their putative role in learning through memory consolidation. An early comparison of sleep architecture of children with reading difficulties with normal children of the same age (8 – 10 years old) showed differences but no special emphasis was placed in spindle activity [109]. A very recent study however comparing Dyslexic and normal children (ages 8 to 16) identified important differences in sleep architecture including an increase in spindle density during NREM 2 [110]. More importantly only the sigma band power in NREM2 was positively correlated with the Word Reading test and in a Memory and Learning Transfer reading test while no significant correlations were found with the Non-Word Reading test; also, a positive significant correlation was found between spindle density and the Word Reading. Although these findings seem to implicate non-rapid eye movement (NREM) sleep and specifically sleep spindles in learning the relation is far from clear and more research is needed.

### 4.5. Spindles in schizophrenia

Recent studies using high-density electroencephalography have revealed a marked reduction in sleep spindles in Schizophrenia. Ferrarelli et al reported using whole-night high-density EEG recordings in 49-schizophrenia patients [111]. They had whole-night deficits in spindle power (12-16Hz) and in slow (12-14 Hz) and fast (14-16 Hz) spindles amplitude, duration, number and integrated spindle activity in prefrontal, centroparietal a d temporal regions. These results indicate that spindle deficits can be reliably established in schizophrenia, are stable across the night, are unlikely to be due to antipsychotic medications, and point to deficit in the thalamic reticular circuits. The reticular thalamic nucleus (TRN) consists of a gamma amino butyric acid (GABA) ergic neurons, which receive excitatory afferents from both cortical and thalamic neurons and sends inhibitory projections to all nuclei of dorsal thalamus.

TRN-thalamus circuits are involved in bottom-up activities, including sensory gating and the transfer to the cortex of sleep spindles. The TRN is implicated in the neurobiology of schizophrenia, the reduction of sleep spindles revealed in schizophrenias, and deficits in attention and sensory gating have been consistently found in Schizophrenia [112]. Schizophrenic patients failed to demonstrate normal sleep-dependent improvement in motor procedural learning. In normal subjects, overnight improvement on the finger tapping motor sequence test (MST) and other simple motor skill tasks specifically correlates with the amount of Stage 2 sleep in the last quartile of the night [113-114]. MST improvement also correlates with number and density of fast spindles [115]. The MST is performed with the left hand, and right>left asymmetry of spindle density and power in the motor cortex observed [114]. Sleep spindles are hypothesized to mediate the consolidation of procedural memory on the MST [114-116] and other motor tasks [64]. However, spindle activity of schizophrenic patients has reduced [117], and s positive relation between stage 2 spindle density and verbal declarative memory performance was observed [118]. In the context of intact practice-dependent learning, chronic medicated schizophrenic patients failed to demonstrate significant overnight improvement of motor procedural memory. They differed significantly from healthy controls, which did show significant improvement. The amount of sleep in the last quartile of the night significantly predicted initial overnight improvement in schizophrenia. The reduction of sleep-dependent consolidation of procedural memory in schizophrenia and sleep makes an important contribution to cognitive deficits [119] and now link variation in the expression of this deficit to specific sleep stages.

## 5. Clinical use of dynamic sleep spindle profiles in organic brain injuries

### 5.1. Sleep, the distribution of spindles, recovery after stroke

The sleep of stroke patients during night time has reported both insomnia and hypersomnia [120]. In the acute stage of hemispheric stroke, poor sleep efficiency [121-122], augmented wakefulness after sleep onset (WASO) [122], increased numbers of awakenings have been reported [123].

Poor sleep efficiency and wakefulness after sleep onset will reduce cognitive function in the acute phase after stroke [124]. Sleep is described as restless, light, or poor-quality sleep, although its duration appears normal.

Spindle distribution may be locally depressed by various types of cortical, subcritical pathology, including the generation of ascending reticular formation and thalamo-cortical pathways. The ipsilateral spindle depression following unilateral frontal leucotomy was first observed [125-126].Cress and Gibbs (1948) observed spindle asymmetries (ipsilateral depression) in 98 % of patients with hemispheric cerebrovascular accidents, whereas only 48% had focal abnormalities in the waking EEG [127].

Many investigations have reported sleep EEG changes following thalamic lesions [128-130].

Such studies may clarify the neuroanatomical circuitry that underlies sleep spindle rhythm generation, and may reveal clinically useful information such as for prognostic purpose or as an objective assessment of recovery from stroke.

Paramedian thalamic stroke (PTS) is an occasional cause of organic hypersomnia, which in the absence of sleep-wake cycle, and has been attributed to disruption of ascending activating impulses and considered a "dearoused "state, the disruption of both arousal and NREM sleep.

A decrease of sleep spindles, slow wave sleep, and REM sleep occurs in patients with the syndrome of fatal thalamic insomnia (FTI), in which neuronal loss is restricted to the anterior and dorsomedial nuclei of the thalamus. Bassetti et al. (1996), reported in 12 patients showed nocturnal polysomnographic findings paralleled the severity of hypersomnia [128]. Hypersomnia following PTS is accompanied by deficient arousal during the day and insufficient spindling and slow wave production at night, The center of the ischemic lesion was the inferior region of dorsomedial nucleus(DM) and the medial anterior part of the CM(centromedian neucles), confirming the autopsy study of Castaine et al [131]. The DM nucleus plays a important role in sleep regulation, and the reduction of spindles and slow-sleep-wave (SWS) was observed, these oscillatory activities are the expressions at neuronal level of different degrees of a same TC neuronal networks. However, an increase of spindles not of SWS suggests that the transition from spindling to SWS depends on the hyper polarization of a critical number of TC neurons.

PET scans showed bilateral thalamic hypometabolism with additional basal ganglia or mesiolateral frontal and cingular hypometabolism in patients with paramedian thalamic calcifications [132]. Wake-sleep studies showed abnormal sleep organization and in the case with frontal and limbic PET hypometabolism ,pre-sleep behaviour associated with "subwakefulness" EEG activities, lack of EEG and spindles and K-complexes, and features of status dissociates. Paramedian thalamic stuructures and interconnected, especially frontal and cingular, areas play a part in the organization of the wake-sleep cycle.

Hermann et al., demonstrated the neurological, neuropsychological, and sleep-wake deficits of 46 paramedian thalamic stroke patients [133]. Oculomotor palsy (76%), mild gait ataxia (67%), deficits of attention (63%), fluency and error control (59%), learning and memory

(67%), and behavior (67%) were common in the acute stroke phase. Outcome was excellent with right-sided infarcts but mostly incomplete with bilateral and left-sided lesions. Long-term recovery after paramedical thalamic stroke is significantly better in right-sided than in bilateral and left-sided. Bilateral and left-sided strokes regularly present with deficits in executive functions and memory, which may persist and will be the unfavorable outcome. Initially, hypersomnia was present in all patients associated with increased stage 1 sleep, reduced stage 2 sleep, and reduced sleep spindles. Post-stroke hypersomnia improves within months, a moderate improvement in sleep spindle activity may occur at the same time, whereas sleep EEG changes may remain unchanged for years.

Further studies are needed to confirm the specificity of these findings for hypersomnia following PTS and to confirm the hypothesis of relationship between spindles, NREM sleep, and cognition.

However there have been few prior studies of the effects of extrathalamic hemispheric lesions on the human sleep EEG. the role of the cerebral hemispheres (cortical, subcortical regions) in the regulation of sleep-wake functions and the modulation of the sleep EEG remains unclear[134]. Physiological experiments with an encephalae isole cat preparation (transected between caudal medulla and spinal cord) established that cortical activation facilitates waking EEG activity due to the presence of corticoreticular projections [135]. The cerebral hemispheres have also been found to contribute to the generation of sleep EEG patterns. The corticothalamic feedback could to support large-scale synchronization of spindle oscillatory activity [136]. Gottselg et al., demonstrated a significant reduction in the power and coherence of sleep spindle activity in EEG recorded over that hemisphere ipsilateral to the lesion during the acute stage of stroke [137]. The cerebral hemispheres are crucially involved in generating synchronous sleep spindles. And they demonstrated that a significant increase in the power and coherence of sleep spindle frequency activity from the acute to the chronic phase of stroke. The plastic mechanism allowed the possibility of recovery to spindle frequency, power and coherence. The stronger ipsilateral effects of cerebral lesions on spindle oscillations indicated reduction of amplitude of sleep spindles in the ipsilateral hemisphere, as well as reduction of cortical activation of spindle oscillations and underling corticothalamic projections [138].

## 5.2. Sleep and the distribution of spindles after traumatic brain injury

Electroencephalographic approach to the clinical assessment of consciousness has been tried in clinical situations with the anticipation that will support the diagnosis and prognosis. Electrical activities of brain tissue to immediately and secondary brain damage have been considered of good prognostic value for brain injury. Many neuroimaging techniques have shown the alterations in the brain parenchyma following severe traumatic brain injury, such as DAI (Diffuse axonal injury), which at the neuronal level, rapid acceleration and deceleration and the consequent rotational forces damage the axons in the cerebral and brain stem white matter, cerebellum. The magnetic resonance imaging (MRI) can show white matter degenerations or small penetrate hemorrhages that normal appearance on CT.

Urakami demonstrated spindle alterations following DAI using simultaneous EEG and MEG recordings [139].

In the postacute stage (mean 80 days) of DAI patients, frequency, amplitude, cortical activation source strength of spindle activities was significantly decreased compared with normal subjects. In the chronic stage (mean 151 days), spindles significantly increased, and no significant difference was found between normal subjects. DAI patients' cognitive functions also improved, with favorable 1-year outcome. Spindle activities may reflect recovery of consciousness, cognitive functions following a DAI [139].

The wide spectrum of sleep disorders in patients with chronic traumatic brain injuries occur, hypersomnia, insomnia, and parasomnia (such as acting out dream, nightmares, sleep paralysis, sleep walking and so on) [140]. Sixty adult patients with TBI, who presented with sleep-related complaints 3 months to 2 years following TBI were analyzed. Sleep disorders are a common finding after the acute phase of TBI. Daytime somnolence may lead to poor daytime performance, altered sleep-wake schedule, heightened anxiety, and poor sense of well being, insomnia and depression. Noticeably, sleep changes and deranged sleep architecture are common in chronic TBI patients. The same as stroke patients, regarding for TBI patients, spindles improve during subacute to chronic stage, while a wide spectrum of sleep disorders remains in chronic stage. Sleep disturbance can compromise the rehabilitation process and the ability to return to work. A diagnosis and subsequent treatment of these disorders may facilitate physical and cognitive rehabilitation of TBI patients.

## 6. Sleep and motor learning

### 6.1. The sleep cycle, memory systems, and memory stages

The human sleep cycle across the night, NREM and REM sleep cycle every 90 min, while the ratio of NREM to REM sleep shifts. During the first half of the night, stages 3 and 4 NREM (SWS) dominate, while stage 2 NREM and REM sleep succeed in the latter half of the night. EEG patterns shows in the different sleep stages, K complexes and sleep spindles occurring during stage 2 NREM, slow (0.5-4 Hz) delta waves developing in slow wave sleep (SWS), and theta waves seen during REM.

Sleep plays an important role in learning process and memory consolidation.

Human memory is divided into declarative forms, with subdivisions into episodic and semantic; and non- declarative forms, subdivided into procedural skill memory [141]. Following the initial encoding of a memory, several ensuring stages are proposed, developing stages of memory, beginning with consolidation, as well as integration of the memory representation, translocation of the representation, during the periods of erasure of the memory. Following later recall, the memory representation is believed to become unstable once again. Memory consolidation refers to a process whereby a memory become increasingly resistant to interference from competing or disrupting factors in absence of further practice [142].

All stages of sleep except sleep onset stage 1 NREM sleep have been implicated in one or more aspects of memory consolidation [143].

Regarding for which stage of sleep is important for the consolidation of a certain memory types, there is some agreement among researchers, however, two different theories exist which explain the role of the various sleep stages on the consolidation of different memory traces [144]. The dual-process theory explains a single sleep stage (REM sleep or SWS) acts and is necessary to form distinct memory traces (procedural or declarative), depending on which memory system that traces is form. The sequential hypothesis, memories are consolidated through the ordered sequence of non-REM sleep followed by REM sleep, so that both stages of sleep are necessary for consolidation. Both non-REM and REM sleep stages, the repeated pattern of non-REM sleep followed by REM sleep are important for memory consolidation. Some memory traces may require more SWS (declarative memory), whereas other memory traces may require more stage 2 non-REM or REM sleep (procedural memory). Rapid eye movement (REM) sleep may be important in processing memory traces and previously learned motor and sensory task. Non-REM (NREM) sleep, particularly slow wave sleep (SWS), its maximal expression in the frontal brain areas, relate to sleep homeostasis and frontal cognitive functions. SWS may increase neuronal plasticity enhancing attention, consolidating procedural and declarative memory [145]. The variability's of the emotional content of the memory, the cognitive weight of the task, and the initial skill level of the learner affect the stage of sleep which concerned the declarative and procedural memory consolidation.

## 6.2. Sleep –dependent memory consolidation

Sleep consolidates new memories by strengthening and integrating them with existing memories. Differentiating sleep-stage specific contributions to neural plasticity as proposed in sleep-dependent memory consolidation. Interest in relationship between mamory consolidation and sleep spindles is comparatively recent. The theories of memory consolidation suggest that storage is initially hippocampally mediated, but gradually gains neocortical representation through dialogue between two structures [146]. Slow oscillations (<1 Hz) allow synchronization between neocortical activity and hippocampal ripples, which are crucial to memory consolidation. Spindles increase during the up-state of slow oscillations [147] and are temporally aligned with hippocampal ripples[148-149],implicating them in the plasticity of hippocampal-neocortical consoridation process. Spindle activity is associated with improvements in procedural and declarative memory [150-152]. Word-pair learning before sleep induced higher sleep spindle activity than a nonlearning task, and spindle activity correlated positively with recall after sleep [153]. Further, Tamminen et al (2010) showed the role of spindles in the integration of newly learned information with existing knowledge, contrasting this with explicit recall of the new information [154]. Spindle activity was associated with overnight lexical integration in the sleep group, but not with gains in recall rate or recognition speed of the novel words themselves. Spindle activity appears to be particularly important for overnight integration of new memories with existing neocortical knowledge.

The strongest functional connectivity between the HF (Hippocampal Formation) (cornu ammonis, dentate gyrus, subiculum)and neocortex was observed in sleep stage 2(compared with both slow-wave sleep) [155]. A strong interaction of sleep spindle occurrence and HF connectivity in sleep stage 2 with increased HF/neocortical connectivity during spindles.

An increase of acetylcholine and a decrease in serotonin during REM sleep in rodents facilitate protein synthesis and long-term potentiation (LTP) in the hippocampus [156]. Both REM sleep and non-REM sleep play a role in long-term synaptic potentiation. Sleep spindles play an important role in sleep-dependent memory improvement. Sleep spindles may depolarize the postsynaptic membrane, resulting in a large influx of calcium ions that leads to cascade of cellular events. These events result in gene expression and protein synthesis necessary for LTP of the postsynaptic membrane.

### 6.3. Sleep promotes motor learning

Sleep following motor skill practice has been demonstrated to enhance motor skill learning off-line (continued overnight improvements in motor skill that are not associated with additional physical practice) for young people who are healthy. However, older adults who are healthy do not benefit from sleep to promote off-line skill enhancement. Patients with chronic stroke demonstrate sleep-dependent off-line motor learning of both implicit and explicit versions of a continuous sequencing task. Sleep enhances both spatial and temporal movement components of a continuous tracking task after stroke. This effect is unique to stroke, age and sex- matched controls that are healthy did not experience sleep- or time-dependent of-line motor learning on either version of the spatial or temporal movement component of task. During the chronic stage of stroke, sleep should be positive between therapy sessions to promote off-line learning of the skill practiced during therapy.

The motor system comprises a network of cortical and subcortical areas interacting by excitatory and inhibitory circuits.

The motor network will be disturbed after stroke when the lesion either directly affects any of these areas or damaged-related white matter tracts. Also abnormal interactions among cortical regions remote from the ischemic lesion might also contribute to the motor impairment after stroke. Pathological intra-and inter-hemispheric interactions among key motor regions constitute an important path pathophysiological aspect of motor impairment after subcortical stroke. Much of the neurobiological mechanisms leading to changes to the changes in cortical connectivity after stroke remain to be elucidated [157].

### 6.4. Sleep-dependent off-line learning in older adults who are healthy

Evidence suggests that stage 2 non-REM sleep, REM sleep or both are associated with consolidation of simple motor task off-line for young people who are healthy. In particular, sleep spindles are an important mechanism of sleep-dependent off-line memory improvement. Sleep-dependent off-line performance enhancement has been conducted using young people who are healthy, and older people are considered not benefit from sleep to enhance motor learning. One hypothesis that older adults fail to demonstrate sleep-dependent off-line motor learning because they experience a reduction in both the time spent in REM sleep and the number of sleep spindles. If older adults who are healthy do not demonstrate sleep-dependent off-line motor learning due to changes in their sleep characteristics, it would follow that altering the sleep characteristics of older adults may enable these individuals to benefit from sleep to enhance off-line motor learning. Increased time spent in REM sleep, greater REM density, and decreased REM latency through the use of sleep-aid medication were correlated with enhanced performance of older adults on a word-recall task [158]. If REM sleep is important for promoting off-line motor learning, older individuals may benefit from sleep to enhance off-line learning if underlying changes in sleep architecture are addressed. Further attempts are required to relate sleep stages and sleep spindles with performance improvement for older people, and potential benefits of modifying these sleep parameters via medication or other means remain to determined.

### 6.5. Sleep-dependent off-line learning after stroke, brain injury

Recent evidence has demonstrated that people with brain injury benefit from sleep to enhance off-line motor learning. Damage to the prefrontal cortex due to stroke, tumor, or trauma demonstrated sleep-dependent off-line learning of a finger sequencing task [159].People with chronic stroke benefit from sleep to enhance motor skill learning of both implicit and explicit versions of a continuous tracking task [160-161]. Sleep also promote off-line motor learning through both improved spatial tracking accuracy and anticipation of upcoming movements in people with chronic stroke [162].A few studies to date have demonstrated the importance of sleep in promoting off-line motor skill learning suggest that stroke or brain injured patients benefit from sleep to enhance off-line learning of motor tasks. Patients with chronic stroke spent about the same amount of time in REM sleep but more time in stage 2 non-REM sleep compared with published norms. The number of sleep spindles increases from acute to chronic stroke. The alterations in sleep architecture demonstrated by chronic stroke patients (maintenance adequate amounts of REM sleep, increase stage 2 non-REM sleep, and increase spindle activity) enable them to demonstrate sleep-dependent skill enhancement. Further works utilizing sleep laboratories is needed to evaluate EEG data and understanding of alterations of sleep architecture and off-line learning of chronic stroke patients.

## 7. Conclusion

### 7.1. Spindles: Outlook and open questions

OQ-1: What is the role of sleep spindles in general and more specifically how do they relate to learning and memory consolidation mechanisms.

OQ-2: What mechanism keeps spindle spectral frequency within so narrow limits, which are stable through the night for a given individual?

OQ-3 related to OQ-2: Why do we observe a step like transition of TC neurons membrane hyperpolarization, which leads from spindles to delta TC rhythm, without appreciable intermediate rhythm frequencies?

QQ-4: How can spindle properties be used as biomarkers for the normal brain function and specific pathological conditions?

## Author details

Yuko Urakami
*National Rehabilitation Center for Persons with Disabilities, Japan*

Andreas A. Ioannides
*Lab. for Human Brain Dynamics, AAI Scientific Cultural Services Ltd., Cyprus*

George K .Kostopoulos
*Dept of Physiology, Medical School, University of Patras, Greece*

## Acknowledgement

The work of YU for this review article was supported by Grants-in-Aid for Scientific Research 23500473 (Japan Society for the Promotion of Science). The work of AAI and GKK was partially funded by the European Commission under the Seventh Framework Programme (FP7/2007-2013) with grant ARMOR, agreement number 287720.

## 8. References

[1] Schomer DL, Lopes da Silva FH.editor. Niedermeyer`s Electroencephalography: Basic Principles, Clinical Applications, and Related Fields. Philadelphia: Lippincott Wiliams & Wilkins; 2010.
[2] Buzsaki G.. editor. Rhythms of the brain, Oxford; 2006.
[3] Gibbs FA, Gibbs EL. Atlas of electroencephalography. Vol.1.Cambridge: Addison-Wesley Press; 1950.
[4] Manshanden I, De Munck JC, Simon NR, Lopes da Silva FH. Source localization of MEG sleep spindles and the relation to sources of alpha band rhythms. Clin Neurophysiol 2002;113(12) 1937-1947.
[5] Urakami Y. Relationships Between Sleep Spindles and Activities of Cerebral Cortex as Determined by Simultaneous EEG and MEG Recording. J Clin Neurophysiol 2008;25(1) 13-24.
[6] Dehghani N, Cash SS, Halgren E. Topographical frequency dynamics within EEG and MEG sleep spindles. Clin Neurophysiol 2011;122(12) 229-235.
[7] Steriade M, McCarley RW. Brain Control of Wakefulness and Sleep. New York: Kluwer Academic;2005.
[8] Kim U, Bal T, McCormick DA. Spindle waves are propagating synchronized oscillations in the ferret LGNd in vitro. J Neurophysiol 1995;74(3) 1301-1323.

[9] Kostopoulos G. Potentiation and modification of recruiting responses precedes the appearance of spike and wave discharges in feline generalized penicillin epilepsy. Electroenceph clin Neurophysiol 1982;53(2) 467-478.

[10] Guillery RW, Feig SL, Lozsadi DA. Paying attention to the thalamic reticular nucleus. Trends Neurosci 1998;21(1) 28-32.

[11] Jones EG. A new view of specific and nonspecific thalamocortical connections. Adv Neurol 1998;77 49-71; discussion 72-73.

[12] Steriade M. Grouping of brain rhythms in corticothalamic systems. Neuroscience 2006;137(4) 1087-1106.

[13] De Gennaro L, Ferrara M. Sleep spindles: an overview. Sleep Med Rev;2003;7(5) 423-440.

[14] Achermann P, Borbély AA. Low-frequency (< 1 Hz) oscillations in the human sleep electroencephalogram. Neuroscience 1997; 81(1) 213-222.

[15] Knoblauch V, Martens WL, Wirz-Justice A, Cajochen C. Human sleep spindle characteristics after sleep deprivation. Clin Neurophysiol 2003;114(12) 2258-2267.

[16] Nuñez A, Curró Dossi R, Contreras D, Steriade M. Intracellular evidence for incompatibility between spindle and delta oscillations in thalamocortical neurons of cat. Neuroscience1992;48(1) 75-85.

[17] Kokkinos V, Kostopoulos GK. Human non-rapid eye movement stage II sleep spindles are blocked upon spontaneous K-complex coincidence and resume as higher frequency spindles afterwards. J Sleep Res 2011;20(1 Pt 1) 57-72.

[18] Paré D, Steriade M, Deschênes M, Oakson G. Physiological characteristics of anterior thalamic nuclei, a group devoid of inputs from reticular thalamic nucleus.J Neurophysiol 1987;57(6) 1669-1685.

[19] Ueda K, Nittono H, Hayashi M, Hori T. Spatiotemporal changes of slow wave activities before and after 14 Hz/12 Hz sleep spindles during stage 2 sleep. Psychiatry Clin Neurosci 2001;55(3) 183-184.

[20] De Gennaro L, Ferrara M. Sleep spindles: an overview. Sleep Med Rev 2003;7(5) 423-440.

[21] Bódizs R, Gombos F, Kovács I. Sleep EEG fingerprints reveal accelerated thalamocortical oscillatory dynamics in Williams syndrome. Res Dev Disabil 2012;33(1) 153-164.

[22] Kolaj M, Zhang L, Rønnekleiv OK, Renaud LP. Midline thalamic paraventricular nucleus neurons display diurnal variation in resting membrane potentials, conductances, and firing patterns in vitro. J Neurophysiol 2012;107(7) 1835-1844.

[23] Jouvet M.,editor. The Paradox of Sleep The Story of Dreaming: MIT Press;1999.

[24] Henri Pieron.,editor. Le problème physiologique du Sommeil. Science 1913; 4,37(953) p525-526. DOI:10.1126/science. 37.953.525,

[25] Kleitman N.The effects of prolonged sleeplessness on man. Am J Physiol 1923;66(1) 67-92.

[26] Aserinsky E, Kleitman N. Regularly Occurring Periods of Eye Motility, and Concomitant Phenomena, During Sleep. Science 1953;118(3062) 273-274.

[27] Hamalainen M, Hari R, Ilmoniemi RJ, Knuutila J, Lounasmaa OV. Magnetoencephalography: theory, instrumentation, and applications to noninvasive studies of the working human brain. Reviews of Modern Physics 1993;65 413-497.

[28] Ioannides AA. Estimates of brain activity using magnetic field tomography and large scale communication within the brain. In: Wan H-M., Popp F-A., Warnke U.(ed.)Bioelectrodynamics and biocommunication.Singapore:World Scientific;1994. p319-353.

[29] Rechtschaffen A., Kales A. editor. A Manual of Standardized Terminology, Techniques and Scoring System for Sleep Stages of Human Subject. Washington DC :US Government Printing Office, National Institute of Health Publication;1968.

[30] Hughes JR, Hendrix DE, Cohen J, Duffy FH, Mayman CI, Scholl ML, Cuffin BN. Relationship of the magnetoencephalogram to the electroencephalogram. Normal wake and sleep activity. Electroencephalogr Clin Neurophysiol 1976;40(3) 261-278.

[31] Yoshida H, Iramina K, Ueno S. Source models of sleep spindles using MEG and EEG measurements. Brain Topogr 1996;8(3) 303-307.

[32] Nakasato N, Kado H, Nakanishi M, Koyanagi M, Kasai N, Niizuma H,Yoshimoto T.Magnetic detection of sleep spindles in normal subjects. Electroencephalogr Clin Neurophysiol 1990;76(2) 123-130.

[33] Lu ST, Kajola M, Joutsiniemi SL, Knuutila S, Hari R. Generator sites of spontaneous MEG activity during sleep. Electroencehalogr Clin Neurophysiol 1992; 82(3) 182-196.

[34] Shih JJ, Weisend MP, Davis JT, Huang M.Magnetoencephalographic characterization of sleep spindles in humans. J Clin Neurophysiol 2000;17(2) 224-231.

[35] Lopes da Silva F. Functional localization of brain sources using EEG and/or MEG data: volume conductor and source models. Magn Reson Imaging 2004;22(10) 1533-1538.

[36] Gumenyuk V, Roth T, Moran JE, Jefferson C, Bowyer SM, Tepley N, Drake CL. Cortical locations of maximal spindle activity: magnetoencephalography (MEG) study. J Sleep Res 2009;18(2) 245-253.

[37] Urakami Y. Relationships Between Sleep Spindles and Activities of Cerebral Cortex as Determined by Simultaneous EEG and MEG Recording. J Clin Neurophysiol 2008; 25(1) 13-24.

[38] Heiss WD, Pawlik G, Herholz K, Wagner R, Wienhard K. Regional cerebral glucose metabolism in man during wakefulness, sleep, and dreaming. Brain Res 1985;327(1-2) 362-366.

[39] Nofzinger EA, Buysse DJ, Miewald JM, Meltzer CC, Price JC, Sembrat RC, Ombao H, Reynolds CF, Monk TH, Hall M, Kupfer DJ, Moore RY. Human regional cerebral glucose metabolism during nonrapid eye movement sleep in relation to waking. Brain 2002; 125(5) 1105-1115.

[40] Picchioni D, Killgore WD, Balkin TJ, Braun AR.Positron emission tomography correlates of visually-scored electroencephalographic waveforms during non-Rapid Eye Movement sleep. Int Neurosci 2009;119(11) 2074-2099.

[41] Allen PJ, Josephs O, Turner R. A Method for Removing Imaging Artifact from Continuous EEG Recorded during Functional MRI. NeuroImage 2000;12(2)230-239.

[42] Schabus M, Dang-Vu TT, Albouy G, Balteau E, Boly M, Carrier J, Desseilles M, Gais S, Phillips C, Rauchs G, Schnakers C, Sterpenich V, Degueldre C, Maquet P. Hemodynamic cerebral correlates of sleep spindles during human non-rapid eye movement sleep. PNAS 2007;104 13164-13169.

[43] Andrade KC, Spoormaker VI, Dresler M, Wehrle R, Holsboer F, Sämann PG, Czisch M. Sleep spindles and hippocampal functional connectivity in human NREM sleep. J Neurosci 2011; 31(28) 10331-10339.

[44] Steriade M, Llinas RR.The functional states of the thalamus and the associated neuronal interplay.Physiol Rev1988; 68 (3) 649-742.

[45] Buzsáki G. The thalamic clock: emergent network properties. Neuroscience1991;41(2-3) 351-364.

[46] Steriade M., editor.The intact and sliced brain. London: MIT Press; 2001.

[47] Andrillon T, Nir Y, Staba RJ, Ferrarelli F, Cirelli C, Tononi G, Fried I. Sleep Spindles in Humans: Insights from Intracranial EEG and Unit Recordings. J Neurosci 2011;31(49) 17821–17834.

[48] Nir Y, Staba RJ, Andrillon T, Vyazovskiy VV, Cirelli C, Fried I,Tononi G. Regional Slow Waves and Spindles in Human Sleep. Neuron 2011;70(1) 153–169.

[49] Terzano MG, Mancia D, Salati MR, Costani G, Decembrino A, Parrino L. The cyclic alternating pattern as a physiologic component of normal NREM sleep. Sleep 1985; 8(2) 137-145.

[50] Ioannides AA, Bolton JPR, Clarke CJS. Continuous probabilistic solutions to the biomagnetic inverse problem. Inverse Probl 1990; 6 523–542.

[51] Pascual-Marqui RD. Review of Methods for Solving the EEG Inverse Problem. Int J Bioelectr 1999;1(1) 75-86. Printed Issue ISSN 1457-7857, Internet Issue ISSN 14567865 (http://www.tut.fi/ijbem).

[52] Ioannides AA. Magnetoencephalography as a research tool in neuroscience: state of the art. Neuroscientist 2006;12(6) 524-544.

[53] Taylor JG, Ioannides AA, MullerGartner HW. Mathematical analysis of lead field expansions.IEEE Trans Med Imaging 1999; 18(2) 151-163.

[54] Ioannides AA, Corsi-Cabrera M, Fenwick PB, del Rio Portilla Y, Laskaris NA, Khurshudyan A, Theofilou D, Shibata T, Uchida S, Nakabayashi T, Kostopoulos GK. MEG tomography of human cortex and brainstem activity in waking and REM sleep saccades. Cereb Cortex 2004;14(1) 56-72.

[55] Ioannides AA, Kostopoulos GK, Liu L, Fenwick PB. MEG identifies dorsal medial brain activations during sleep. Neuroimage 2009;44(2) 455-468.

[56] Koenigs M, Holliday J, Solomon J, Grafman J. Left Dorsomedial Frontal Brain Damage Is Associated with Insomnia. J Neurosci 2010;30(41) 16041-16043.

[57] Ioannides AA, Liu L, Urakami Y, Kostopoulos GK. Spindles and activity in the spindle frequency range during stage 2 sleep.2012 (Human Brain Mapping Abstract, Beijing 2012).

[58] Anderer P, Klösch G, Gruber G, Trenker E, Pascual-Marqui RD, Zeitlhofer J, Barbanoj MJ, Rappelsberger P, Saletu B. Low-resolution brain electromagnetic tomography

revealed simultaneously active frontal and parietal sleep spindle sources in the human cortex. Neurosci 2001;103(3) 581-592.

[59] Ventouras E, Ktonas PE, Tsekou H, Paparrigopoulos T, Kalatzis I,Sldatos CR. Independent component analysis for source lacalization of EEG sleep spindle components.Comput Intell Neurosci 2010; 329436. Epub 2010 Mar 29.

[60] Dehghani N, Cash SS, Chen CC, Hagler DJ Jr, Huang M, Dale AM, Halgren E. Divergent cortical generators of MEG and EEG during human sleep spindles suggested by distributed source modeling. PLoS One 2010;5(7) e11454.

[61] Dehghani N, Cash SS, Halgren E. Topographical frequency dynamics within EEG and MEG sleep spindles. Clin Neurophysiol 2011;122(2) 229-235.

[62] Dehghani N, Cash SS,Halgren E.Emergence of synchronous EEG spindles from asynchronous MEG spindles. Hum Brain Mapp 2011;32(12) 2217-2227.

[63] Schabus M, Hodlmoser K, Gruber G, Sauter C, Anderer P, Klosch G, Parapatics S, Saletu B, Klimesch W, Zeitlhofer J. Sleep spindle-related activity in the human EEG and its relation to general cognitive and learning abilities Eur J Neurosci 2006;23(7) 1738-1746.

[64] Tamaki M, Matsuoka T, Nittono H, Hori T.Fast sleep spindle (13–15 Hz) activity correlates with sleep-dependent improvement in visuomotor performance. Sleep 2008;31(2) 204-211.

[65] Steriade M, McCarley RW.,editors. Brain Control of Wakefulness and Sleep. New York: Kluwer Academic;2005.

[66] Jankel WR, Niedermeyer E. Sleep spindles. J Clin Neurophysiol 1985;2(1) 1-35.

[67] Schabus M, Dang-Vu TT, Heib DP, Boly M, Desseilles M, Vandewalle G, Schmidt C, Albouy G, Darsaud A, Gais S, Degueldre C, Balteau E, Phillips C, Luxen A, Maquet P. The Fate of Incoming Stimuli during NREM Sleep is Determined by Spindles and the Phase of the Slow Oscillation. Front Neurol 2012;3(40).

[68] Himanen SL,Virkkala J, Huhtala H. Spindle frequencies in sleep EEG show U-shape within first four NREM sleep episodes. J Sleep Res 2002; 11(1) 35-42.

[69] Kostopoulos GK. Involvement of the thalamocortical system in epileptic loss of consciousness. Epilepsia 2001;42 Suppl 3 S13-S19.

[70] Hofle N, Paus T, Reutens D, Fiset P, Gotman J, Evans AC,Jones BE. Regional Cerebral Blood Flow Changes as a Function of Delta and Spindle Activity during Slow Wave Sleep in Humans. J Neurosci 1997;17(12) 4800-4808.

[71] Kokkinos V, Kostopoulos GK.Human non-rapid eye movement stage II sleep spindles are blocked upon spontaneous K-complex coincidence and resume as higher frequency spindles afterwards. J Sleep Res 2011;20(1 Pt 1) 57-72.

[72] Tononi G. Information integration: its relevance to brain function and consciousness. Arch Ital Biol 2010;148(3) 299-322.

[73] Kostopoulos GK. Recent advances in sleep physiology of interest to psychoanalysis. International Forum of Psychoanalysis.2012; 22 1-10.

[74] Franks NP. General anaesthesia: from molecular targets to neuronal pathways of sleep and arousal. Nat Rev Neurosci 2008; 9(5) 370-386.

[75] Cologan V, Schabus M, Ledoux D, Moonen G, Maquet P, Laureys S. Sleep in disorders of consciousness. Sleep Med Rev 2010;14(2) 97-105.

[76] Loeb C, Poggio GF. Electroencephalogram in a case with pontomesencephalic hemorrhage. Electroencephalogr Clin Neurophysiol1953;5(2) 295-296.

[77] Jasper HH, Van Buren J.Interrelationship between cortex and subcortical structures: clinical electroencephalographic studies. Electroencephalogr Clin Neurophysiol 1955;Suppl 4 S168-S188.

[78] Hughes JR,Cayaffa J, Leestma J. Electro-clinical pathologic correlations in comatose patients.Clin Electroencephalogr 1976;7 13-30.

[79] Steudel WI, Krüger J, Grau H. Zur Alpha-und Spindel-Activität bei komatosen Patienten nach einer Schädel-Hirn –Vertetzung unter besonderer Berücksichtigung der Computertomographie.Z EEG-EMG 1979;10 143-147.

[80] Silverman D. Retrospective study of EEG in coma. Electroencephalogr Clin Neurophysiol 1963;15 486-503.

[81] Rumpl E, Prugger M, Bauer F, Gerstenbrand F, Hackl JM,Pallua A. Incidence and prognosis value of spindles in post-traumatic coma. Electroencephalogr Clin Neurophysiol 1983;56(5) 420-429.

[82] Britt CW Jr. Nontraumatic "spindle coma": clinical, EEG, and prognostic features. Neurology1981; 31(4)393-397.

[83] Britt CW Jr, Raso E, Gerson LP. Spindle coma, secondary to primary traumatic midbrain hemorrhage. Electroencephalogr Clin Neurophysiol 1980;49(3-4) 406-408.

[84] Seet RC, Lim EC, Wilder-Smith EP. Spindle coma from acute midbrain infarction. Neurology 2005; 64(12) 2159-2160.

[85] Kotagal P, Yardi N. The relationship between sleep and epilepsy. Semin Pediatr Neurol 2008;15(2) 42-49.

[86] Kostopoulos GK. Brain Mechanisms Linking Epilepsy to Sleep. In: Philip A. Schwartzkroin.(ed.) Encyclopedia of Basic Epilepsy Research 3.Oxford: Academic Press;2009.p1327-1336.

[87] Matos G,Tufik S,Scorza FA, Cavalheiro EA, Andersen ML. Sleep, epilepsy, and translational research: what can we learn from laboratory bench? Prog Neurobiol 2011;95(3) 396-405.

[88] Asano E, Mihaylova T, Juhász C, Sood S,Chugani HT. Effect of sleep on interictal spikes and distribution of sleep spindles on electrocorticography in children with focal epilepsy.Clin Neurophysiol 2007;118(6) 1360-1368.

[89] Panayiotopoulos CP., editor. The epilepsies: seizures, syndromes and management. Oxford:Bladon Medical Publishing;2005.

[90] Kellaway P, Frost JD, Crawley JW. The relationship between sleep spindles and spike-and-wave bursts in human epilepsy. In Avoli M., Gloor P., Kostopoulos G., Naquet R. (ed.) Generalized epilepsy: neurobiological approaches, Boston: Birkhauser;1990. p36-48.

[91] Gloor P. Generalized epilepsy with bilateral synchronous spike and wave discharge. New findings concerning its physiological mechanism.Electroencephalogr Clin Neurophysiol 1978;Suppl 34 S245-S249.

[92] Avoli M. A brief history on the oscillating roles of thalamus and cortex in absence seizures. Epilepsia 2012;53(5)779-789.

[93] Kostopoulos GK. Spike-and-wave discharges of absence seizures as a transformation of sleep spindles: the continuing development of a hypothesis. Clin Neurophysiol 2000;111Suppl 2 S27-S38.

[94] Avanzini G, Vergnes M, Spreafico R, Marescaux C. Calcium dependent regulation of genetically determined spike and waves by the reticular thalamic nucleus of rats. Epilepsia1993;34(1) 1-7.

[95] McCormick DA, Contreras D. On the cellular and network bases of epileptic seizures. Annu Rev Physiol2001; 63 815-846.

[96] van Luijtelaar G, Sitnikova E. Global and focal aspects of absence epilepsy: the contribution of genetic models. Neurosci Biobehav Rev 2006;30(7) 983-1003.

[97] Leresche N, Lambert RC, Errington AC, Crunelli V. From sleep spindles of natural sleep to spike and wave discharges of typical absence seizures: is the hypothesis still valid? Pflugers Arch 2012;463(1) 201-212.

[98] Kostopoulos G, Gloor P, Pellegrini A, Gotman J. A study of the transition from spindles to spike and wave discharge in feline generalized penicillin epilepsy: microphysiological features. Exp Neurol 1981;73(1) 55-77.

[99] Gloor P, Pellegrini A, Kostopoulos GK. Effects of changes in cortical excitability upon the epileptic bursts in generalized penicillin epilepsy of the cat. Electroencephalogr Clin Neurophysiol 1979; 46(3) 274-289.

[100] Gloor P, Avoli M, Kostopoulos G.Thalamocortical relationships in generalized epilepsy with bilaterally synchronous spike-and-wave discharge. In Avoli M., Gloor P., Kostopoulos G., Naquet R. (ed.) Generalized epilepsy: neurobiological approaches. Boston: Birkhauser;1990.p190-212.

[101] Amor F, Baillet S, Navarro V, Adam C, Martinerie J, Quyen MV. Cortical local and long-range synchronization interplay in human absence seizure initiation. Neuroimage 2009;45(3) 950-962.

[102] Stefan H, Paulini-Ruf A, Hopfengärtner R, Rampp S. Network characteristics of idiopathic generalized epilepsies in combined MEG/EEG. Epilepsy Res 2009; 85(2-3) 187-198.

[103] Tucker DM, Brown M, Luu P, Holmes MD. Discharges in ventromedial frontal cortex during absence spells. Epilepsy Behav 2007;11(2-3) 546-557.

[104] Westmijse I, Ossenblok P, Gunning B, van Luijtelaar G. Onset and propagation of spike and slow wave discharges in human absence epilepsy: A MEG study. Epilepsia 2009;50(12) 2538-2548.

[105] Bai X,Vestal M,Berman R,Negishi M,Spann M,Vega C,Desalvo M, Novotny EJ,Constable RT,Blumenfeld H. Dynamic time course of typical childhood absence seizures: EEG, behavior, and functional magnetic resonance imaging. J Neurosci 2010; 30(17) 5884-5893.

[106] Moeller F, LeVan P, Muhle H, Stephani U, Dubeau F, Siniatchkin M, Gotman J. Absence seizures: individual patterns revealed by EEG-fMRI. Epilepsia 2010;51(10) 2000-2010.

[107] Bonakis A, Koutroumanidis M.Epileptic discharges and phasic sleep phenomena in patients with juvenile myoclonic epilepsy. Epilepsia 2009;50(11) 2434-2445.

[108] Koutroumanidis M,Tsiptsios D,Kokkinos V,Kostopoulos GK.Focal and generalized EEG paroxysms in childhood absence epilepsy: Topographic associations and distinctive behaviors during the first cycle of non-REM sleep. Epilepsia 2012; 53(5) 840-849.

[109] Mercier L, Pivik RT,Busby K. Sleep patterns in reading disabled children. Sleep1993;16(3) 207-215.

[110] Bruni O, Ferri R, Novelli L, Terribili M, Trianiello M, Finotti E,Leuzzi V,Curatolo P. Sleep spindle activity is correlated with reading abilities in developmental dyslexia. Sleep 2009; 32(10) 1333-1340.

[111] Ferrarelli F, Peterson MJ, Sarasso S, Brady A, Riedner BA, Michael J, Murphy BS, Benca RM, Bria P, Kalin NH, Tononi G. Thalamic dysfunction in schizophrenia suggested by whole-night deficits in slow and fast spindles. Am J Psychiatr 2012;167 (11) 1339-1348.

[112] Ferrarelli F, Tononi G. The thalamic reticular nucleus and schizophrenia. Schizophr Bull 2011;37(2) 306-315.

[113] Fogel SM, Nader R, Cote KA, Smith CT. Sleep spindles and learning potential. Behav Neurosci 2007;121(1) 1-10.

[114] Walker MP, Brakefield T, Morgan A, Hobson JA, Stickgold R. Practice with sleep makes perfect: sleep-dependent motor skill leaning. Neuron 2002;35(1) 205-211.

[115] Rasch B, Pommer J, Diekelmann S, Born J. Pharmacological REM sleep suppression paradoxically improves rather than impairs skill memory. Nat Neurosci 2009;12(4) 396-397.

[116] Nishida M, Walker MP. Daytime naps, motor memory consolidation and regionally specific sleep spindles. PLoS One 2007;2(4) 341-347.

[117] Ferrarelli F, Huber R, Peterson MJ, Massimini M, Murphy M, Riedner BA. Reduced sleep spindle activity in schizophrenia patients. Am J Psychiatr 2007;164 483-492.

[118] Goder R, Fritzer G, Gottwald B, Lippmann B, Seeck-Hirschner M, Serafin I, Aldenhoff JB. Effects of olanzapine on slow wave sleep, spindles and sleep-related memory consolidation in schizophrenia. Pharmacopsychiatry 2008;41(3) 92-99.

[119] Manoach DS, Katharine N, Thakkar ES, Alice E, Sophia KM, Erin W, Djonlagic I, Vangel MG, Goff DC, Stickgold R. Reduced overnight consolidation of procedural learning in chronic medicated schizophrenia is related to specific sleep stages. J Psychiatr Res 2010;44(2) 112-120.

[120] Bakken LN, Lee KA, Kim HS, Finset A, Lerdal A. Sleep-wake patterns during the acute phase after first-ever stroke. Stroke Res Treat 2011; 936298.

[121] Hachinski VC.Sleep morphology and prognosis in acute cerebrovascular lesions. In: Meyer J., Lechner H., Reivich M. (ed.) Cerebral vascular disease. Amsterdam: Excerpta Medica;1977.p69-71.

[122] Körner E, Flooh E, Reinhart B, Wolf R, Ott E, Krenn W, Lechner H. Sleep alterations in ischemic stroke. Eur Neurol 1986; 25 Suppl 2 104-110.

[123] Giubilei F, Iannilli M, Vitale A, Pierallini A, Sacchetti ML, Antonini G, Fieschi C.Sleep patterns in acute ischemic stroke. Acta Neurol Scand 1992; 86(6) 567-571.

[124] Siccoli MM, Rolli-Baumeler N, Achermann P,Bassetti CL. Correlation between sleep and cognitive functions after hemispheric ischaemic stroke. Eur J Neurol 2008;15(6) 565-572.

[125] Lennox MA, Coolidge J. Electroencephalographic changes after prefrontal lobectomy. Arch Neurol Psychiatry 1949; 62. 150-161.

[126] Kruger EG, Wayne HL. Clinical and electroencephalographic effects of prefrontal lobectomy and lobectomy in chronic psychosis.Arch Neurol Psychiatry1952;67 661-671.

[127] Cress CH, Gibbs EL. Electroencephalographic asymmetry during sleep in patients with vascular and traumatic hemiplegia. Dis Nerv Syst 1948; 9(11) 327-329.

[128] Bassetti C, Mathis J, Gugger M, Lovblad KO, Hess CW. Hypersomnia following paramedian thalamic stroke: a report of 12 patients. Ann Neurol 1996; 39(4) 471-480.

[129] Roth C, Jeanmonod D, Magnin M, Morel A, Achermann P. Effects of medial thalamotomy and pallido-thalamic tractotomy on sleep and waking EEG in pain and Parkinsonian patients. Clin Neurophysiol 2000;111(7) 1266-1275.

[130] Santamaria J, Pujol M, Orteu N, Solanas A, Cardenal C, Santacruz P,Chimeno E, Moon P. Unilateral thalamic stroke does not decrease ipsilateral sleep spindles. Sleep 2000;23(3) 333-339.

[131] Castaigne P, Lhermitte F, Buge A, Escourdolle R, Hauw JJ, Lyon-Caen O. Paramedian thalamic and midbrain infarcts: clinical and neuropathological study. Ann Neurol 1981;10(2) 127-148.

[132] Montagna P, Provini F,Plazzi G, Vetrugno R, Gallassi R, Pierangeli G, Ragno M, Cortelli P, Perani D. Bilateral paramedian thalamic syndrome: abnormal circadian wake-sleep and autonomic functions. J Neurol Neurosurg Psychiatry 2002; 73(6) 772-774.

[133] Hermann DM, Siccoli M, Brugger P,Wachter K, Mathis J, Achermann P,Bassetti CL. Evolution of Neurological, Neuropsychological and Sleep-Wake Disturbances After Paramedian Thalamic Stroke. Stroke 2008;39(1) 62-68.

[134] Jones BE. Basic mechanisms of sleep-wake states. In: Kryger MH., Roth T., Dement WC.(ed.) Principle and practice of sleep medicine. Philadelphia: W.B. Saunders; 2000; 134-154.

[135] Bremer F, Terzuolo C. Contribution à l'étude des méchanismes physiologique du maintien de l'activité vigile du cerveau. Interaction de la formation réticulée et de l'écorce cérébrale dans le processus du réveil. Arch Int Physiol 1954;62(2) 157-178.

[136] Destexhe A, Contreras D, Steriade M. Mechanisms underlying the synchronizing action of corticothalamic feedback through inhibition of thalamic relay cells. J Neurophysiol 1998;79(2) 999-1016.

[137] Gottselig JM, Bassetti CL, Achermann P. Power and coherence of sleep spindle frequency activity following hemispheric stroke. Brain 2002;125(Pt 2) 373-383.

[138] Urakami Y. Relationships between sleep spindles and activities of the cerebral cortex after hemispheric stroke as determined by simultaneous EEG and MEG recordings. J Clin Neurophysiol 2009; 26(4) 248-256.

[139] Urakami Y. Relationships between sleep spindles and clinical outcome in patients with traumatic brain injury: a simultaneous EEG and MEG study. Clin EEG Neurosci 2012;43(1) 39-47.

[140] Verma A, Anand V,Verma NP. Sleep disorders in chronic traumatic brain injury. J Clin Sleep Med 2007; 3(4) 357-362.

[141] Squire LR, Wixted JT. The cognitive neuroscience of human memory since H.M. Annu Rev Neurosci 2011;34 259-288.

[142] McGaugh JL. Memory: a century of consolidation. Science 2000;287(5451) 248-251.

[143] Rauchs G, Desgranges B, Foret J, Eustache F. The relationships between memory systems and sleep stages. J Sleep Res 2005;14(2) 123-140.

[144] Siengsukon CF, Boyd LA. Sleep to learn after stroke: implicit and explicit off-line motor learning. Neurosci Lett 2009; 451(1) 1-5.

[145] Walker MP, Stickgold R. Sleep-dependent learning and memory consolidation. Neuron 2004;44(1) 121-133.

[146] Buzsáki G. Memory consolidation during sleep : a neurophysiological perspective. J Sleep Res 1998; 7 Suppl 1 S17-S23.

[147] Mölle M, Marshall L, Gais S, Born J. Grouping of spindle activity during slow oscillations in human non-rapid eye movement sleep. J Neurosci 2002;22(24) 10941-10947.

[148] Siapas AG, Wilson MA. Coordinated interactions between hippocampal ripples and cortical spindles during slow-wave sleep. Neuron 1998; 21(5) 1123-1128.

[149] Sirota A, Csicsvari J, Buhl D, Buzsáki G. Communication between neocortex and hippocampus during sleep in rodents. Proc Natl Acad Sci USA. 2003;100(4) 2065-2069.

[150] Schabus M, Gruber G, Parapatics S, Sauter C, Klosch G, Anderer P, Klimesch W, Saletu B, Zeitlhofer J. Sleep spindles and their significance for declarative memory consolidation. Sleep 2004;27(8) 1479-1485.

[151] Clemens Z, Fabó D, Halász P. Overnight verbal retention correlates with the number of sleep spindles. Neuroscience 2005; 132(2) 529-535.

[152] Schmidt C, Peigneux P, Muto V, Schenkel M, Knoblauch V, Munch M, de Quervain DJ, Wirz-Justice A,Cajochen C. Encoding difficulty promotes postlearning changes in sleep spindle activity during napping. J Neurosci 2006;26(35) 8976-8982.

[153] Gais S, Molle M, Helms K, Born J. Learning-dependent increases in sleep spindle density. J Neurosci 2002;22(15) 6830-6834.

[154] Tamminen J, Payne JD, Stickgold R, Wamsley EJ, Gaskell MG. Sleep Spindle Activity is Associated with the Integration of New Memories and Existing Knowledge. J Neurosci 2010; 30(43): 14356-14360.

[155] Andrade KC, Spoormaker VI, Dresler M, Wehrle R, Holsboer F, Sämann PG, Czisch M. Sleep Spindles and Hippocampal Functional Connectivity in Human NREM Sleep. J Neurosci 2011;31(28) 10331-10339.

[156] Graves L. Pack A, Abel T. Sleep and memory: a molecular perspective.Trends Neurosci 2001;24(4) 237-243.

[157] Grefkes C, Fink GR. Reorganization of cerebral networks after stroke: new insights from neuroimaging with connectivity approaches.Brain 2011;134(Pt 5) 1264-1276.

[158] Schredl M, Weber B, Leins ML, Heyser I. Donepazil-induced REM sleep augmentation enhances memory performance in eldery,healthy persons. Exp Gerontol 2001;36(2) 353-361.

[159] Gomez Beldarrain M, Astorgano AG., Gonzalez AB.Garcia-Monco JC. Sleep improves sequential motor learning and performance in patients with prefrontal lobe lesions. Clin Neurol Neurosurg 2008;110(3) 245-252.

[160] Siengsukon CF, Boyd LA. Sleep to learn after stroke: implicit and explicit off-line motor learning. Neurosci Lett 2009;451(1) 1-5.

[161] Siengsukon CF, Boyd LA.Sleep enhances implicit motor skill learning in individuals post-stroke. Top Stroke Rehabil 2008;15(1) 1-12.

[162] Siengsukon CF, Boyd LA. Does Sleep Promote Motor Learning? Implications for Physical Rehabilitation. Physical Therapy 2009;89(4) 370-383.

Chapter 5

# Neuromuscular Disorders in Critically-Ill Patients – Approaches to Electrophysiologic Changes in Critical Illness Neuropathy and Myopathy

Fariba Eslamian and Mohammad Rahbar

Additional information is available at the end of the chapter

http://dx.doi.org/10.5772/50543

## 1. Introduction

Neurologic causes of profound weakness in an ICU (Intensive Care Unit) patient include disorders of the central nervous system (CNS) and the peripheral nervous system (PNS). Some of these are primary neurologic disorders that result in admission to the ICU, whereas others occur while the patient experiences prolonged hospitalization for unrelated medical problems.

These numerous non neurologic medical causes mainly including ischemic or hemorrhagic strokes, respiratory failure followed by COPD (chronic obstructive pulmonary disease) and asthma, acute or chronic renal failure, complications of ischemic heart diseases such as myocardial infarction and consequences of malignant processes. Most of these patients undergo mechanical ventilation, some of whom would subsequently be affected by neuromuscular disorders.

From the point of view of electroneurophysiology, these disorders are divided into three categories: 1) Critical Illness Neuropathy (CIN), 2) Critical Illness Myopathy (CIM), and 3) Prolonged Neuromuscular Junction Blockage [1].

In the present chapter, all of three above mentioned disorders as well as two axonal variants of Guillain-Barré Syndrome (GBS), namely Acute Motor Axonal Neuropathy (AMAN) and Acute Motor and Sensory Axonal Neuropathy (AMSAN) will be discussed in detail, which have differential diagnostic importance in distinguishing the etiology of weakness in critically-ill patients. Furthermore, we would have a glimpse into our experience derived from 14 hospitalized patients with prominent clinical picture of profound weakness, studying and comparing their neuromuscular disorders as clinical, electrodiagnostic, underlying diseases and incidence rate aspects, individually.

## 2. Clinical presentation

Major clinical manifestation of these disorders includes a progressive weakness of the upper and lower extremities or all four limbs as quadriplegia or paraplegia along with hyporeflexia, hypotonia, with or without atrophy and weakness of the respiratory muscles.

The most common scenario commence with ICU hospitalization of the patients due to serious non-neurological medical reasons including above-mentioned etiologies (renal failure, COPD exacerbation, cerebral and gastrointestinal hemorrhage etc.). Majority of these patients are dependent on the ventilator and require neuromuscular junction blocking agents (NMBAs). During the recovery phase, the focus is on tapering sedatives and NMBAs which could be associated with occurrence of flaccid weakness in the upper and lower extremities and respiratory muscles; this in turns would delay weaning process from the ventilator [2]. On the other hand, patient status is likely to deteriorate toward sepsis or multi-organ failure and becoming ventilator-dependent for a long time. Performing electrodiagnostic tests to detect neuromuscular disorders delaying extubation is, hence, highly-indicated at this stage.

### 2.1. Electrodiagnostic studies in ICU patients, technical issues

Although electrodiagnostic (EDX) studies are mainly performed in outpatient setting, the number of the EDX studies in inpatient setting or hospitalized patients in ICU has recently been increased [2]. There is a number of challenging technical issues unique to performing EDX studies in the ICU and complicated ill patients. Some are related to patient factors, whereas others involve central and intravenous lines and electrical equipment that interfere with the performance of the study.

As previously mentioned, in these cases patients are profoundly ill, often with several serious overlapping medical problems. Most are intubated and receiving mechanical ventilation, which prevents them from traveling to the EMG laboratory, necessitating a portable study. But portable EDX device has its own problems such as interference with other electrical devices attached to the patient in ICU, noise and artifact production and increasing the potential risk of an electrical injury for sensitive patients.

These patients are often poorly cooperative and heavily sedated or agitated, who would not be able to roll on the sides or maintain positions required for performing the sensory or motor electrodiagnostic tests. Neither the agitated patient nor the sedated patient is able to give the electromyographer proper feedback during the study, for example, whether he or she is feeling the stimulus during the nerve conduction studies. Nor can such patients place their limbs in the correct position for the nerve conduction studies or the spontaneous activity assessment portion of the needle examination. Finally, they cannot cooperate with the examiner to activate their muscles voluntarily when trying to assess motor unit action potentials (MUAPs) during the needle examination [2].

## 3. Our study patients

Fourteen hospitalized patients from the Pulmonology ICU, Neurology and Internal Medicine wards with primary or secondary progressive weakness of the upper and lower limbs with or without respiratory muscles involvement were referred to the electrodiagnostic center, Physical Medicine and Rehabilitation department, Imam Reza Hospital, Tabriz, Iran in a one and half year period from August 2010 to February 2012.

In order to evaluate neuromuscular disorders and to diagnose the causes of weakness electro-neurophysiologically, Nerve Conduction Study and Needle Electromyography (NCS-EMG) were performed in all of referred patients. The data related to these patients including age, sex, admission reason, underlying diseases, past medical history, final diagnosis ,treatments and outcome are presented in Table-1.

A total of 14 patients were selected and examined. Based on NCS-EMG studies, patients were diagnosed as CIN in 4, CIM in 3, neuromyopathic critical illness in 4; including two patients with a combination of CIM and CIN and other two patients with previous acute or chronic neuropathy and superimposed subsequent CIM, AMAN in 2 and AMSAN only in one patient. We would briefly discuss about clinical and electrodiagnostic principals, techniques and features each of these entities in the next sections.

## 4. Critical Illness Neuropathy (CIN)

CIN or CIP (Critical Illness Polyneuropathy) is reported as the most common severe neuropathy in ICU patients, mostly observed in patients hospitalized due to primary non-neurological medical problems. The main reason for its occurrence is a reactive systemic inflammatory response to sepsis or trauma [2]. Unlike GBS, CIN is an axonal polyneuropathy and considered whenever there are signs of fixed weakness in the extremities, sensory loss or inability to wean from the ventilator despite beginning clinical improvement of the patient.

Although CIN has been reported to be more frequent than CIM in several studies [3], in a study with 88 patients, the incidence ratio of CIM was reported to be three times more than CIN (42% vs. 13%). The results of this study showed that among patients who underwent EMG in ICU population, acute myopathy is three times as common as acute axonal polyneuropathy, and the outcomes from acute myopathy and acute axonal polyneuropathy may be similar [4]. In other words, mortality and morbidity are comparable in both of them.

In addition to polyneuropathy, mononeuropathies including unilateral or bilateral phrenic neuropathy are frequently seen in CIN, which contribute to respiratory disorders requiring EDX for accurate diagnosis [2].

### 4.1. Electrophysiologic features in CIN

Although, as above mentioned, EDX is associated with difficulties in ill and complicated patients, based on previous studies as well as present study results, electrodiagnostic findings could be summarized as the following:

Compound muscle action potentials (CMAPs) are profoundly reduced in amplitude or absent. Motor conduction velocities are normal or slightly reduced and distal latencies are normal or slightly prolonged, while sensory nerve action potentials (SNAPs) should be significantly diminished in amplitude or unobtainable. Phrenic nerve study also reveals absence or reduction of obtained CMAP from diaphragm muscle, which will be explained in the end of this section.

In pure CIN, neurogenic pattern including high amplitude and polyphasic motor unit action potentials (MUAPs) with reduced recruitment are observed in needle electromyography [5]. However, patients are sometimes unable to perform motor units recruitment and nothing could be detected due to patients' poor effort. In these situations, the only observable sign in the needle EMG would be presence of denervation potentials (fib/psw) at the rest phase of needle exam.

Electrodiagnostic criteria of the present study were based on these principals and all of above-mentioned characteristics were applied to our patients diagnosed with CIN as well.

Some points should be highlighted regarding the EDX findings in CIN: *firstly,* if SNAPs were normal or mildly low amplitude associated with diminished CMAPs, other diagnosis rather than CIN would be investigated i.e. CIM (critical illness myopathy) or AMAN (motor axonal neuropathy). At this point, needle EMG differentiates these two entities from each other. *Secondly,* another fact to be kept in mind is that low amplitude SNAPs could be related to previous underlying disease such as diabetes or renal failure and subsequent diabetic or uremic neuropathy rather than CIN. *Thirdly,* in cases with mixed CIN and CIM, in spite of the fact that SNAPs are abnormal, myogenic pattern in needle EMG demonstrates muscle weakness may be more related to the superimposed myopathy.

## 4.2. Phrenic nerve electrodiagnostic study

One of the major reasons contributing to unsuccessful weaning trials from the ventilator in intubated patients is unilateral or bilateral phrenic neuropathy which could be idiopathic, due to autoimmune or post-infection etiologies such as Bell's palsy and secondary to iatrogenic causes after coronary artery bypass grafting or other thoracic surgeries [2].

Phrenic nerve could also be affected as an accompanying disorder observed with polyneuropathies such as GBS or CIN. To obtain phrenic nerve CMAP, recording electrode is secured a few centimeters proximal to the xyphoid process while the reference electrode being placed 16 cm lower along with the ribcage on both sides corresponding to the phrenic nerve excited. Stimulation electrode is placed 3 cm superior to the clavicle parallel to the cricoid cartilage [6]. The important issue is that normal amplitude for phrenic CMAP is 300-500 μv which in fact could be associated with unclear responses due to the electrical noise existing in the ICU.

| No. of Patients | Age | sex | The cause of admission | Underlying disease | Past Medical History | Progress of disease and outcome | Electrodiagnostic Impression |
|---|---|---|---|---|---|---|---|
| # 1 | 64 | M | Respiratory failure | gastric cancer | Surgery of total Gastrectomy, IHD,Asthma | Mechanical ventilation, worsening of general status ,expire | CIN[a] |
| # 2 | 63 | F | Acute pancreatitis | - | - | Treatment of pancreatitis and recovery | CIN |
| # 3 | 36 | M | Acute Respiratory distress Syndrome (ARDS) | Methadone poisoning | Addiction | GI bleeding, hypoxic Encephalopathy+ Intubation | CIN |
| # 4 | 66 | M | Acute renal failure (ARF) | ATN[b] secondary to over dosage of NSAIDs | NSAIDs intake because of musculoskeletal problems | Treatment of Pneumonia, Hemodialysis for ARF, recovery | CIN |
| # 5 | 15 | F | Rectal bleeding and unconsciousness | Seliac disease | Surgery of Appendectomy | Bowel obstruction, respiratory disturbance +intubation | CIM[C] |
| # 6 | 37 | M | Dyspenea exacerbation | corpulmonale | Kyphoscoliosis in thoracic and lumbar spinal area | Mechanical ventilation + tracheostomy, partial recovery | CIM |
| # 7 | 54 | F | Intra ventricular hemorrhage (IVH) | ICH[d], IVH and hydrocephaly | Hypertension | Intubation+ prolonged Mechanical ventilation, expire | CIM |
| # 8 | 66 | M | Dyspenea exacerbation | COPD [e] | COPD, Diabetes, hypertension | Intubation+ prolonged Mechanical ventilation | CIN/CIM [f] |
| # 9 | 25 | M | quadriparesia | Traumatic SCI in C5-C6 levels | - | Prominent LMN[g] signs (Lower and upper limbs weakness, hypotonia and hyporeflexia),excess of UMN[h] signs related to SCI | CIN/CIM |
| # 10 | 55 | M | Progressive lower limbs weakness | LBP | History of LBP, radiculopathy, epidural injections | Treatment for neuropathy and CIM, partial recovery | CIM super-imposed on chronic sensorimotor polyneuro-pathy |
| # 11 | 42 | F | Progressive lower and upper limbs weakness | FUO (fever with unknown origin) | First admission 40 days before second admission, because of FUO and then treatment for GBS | Treatment for tuberculosis meningitis ,treatment for following AMAN and CIM, partial recovery with persistent paraparesia | CIM, superimposed on AMAN[I] |
| # 12 | 44 | F | Progressive lower limbs weakness | Lumbar radiculopathy | LBP and history of lumbar disc surgery three months ago. | Complicated with pulmonary thrombo emboli (PTE), phrenic nerve neuropathy | AMAN |
| # 13 | 72 | M | Progressive lower limbs weakness | Upper respiratory infection | Weakness started one week after respiratory infection | Treatment for AMAN with IVIG and recovery | AMAN |
| # 14 | 60 | M | Exacerbation of COPD | COPD | COPD | 2 weeks after admission lower limbs weakness was occurred, treatment for COPD and following AMSAN | AMSAN[J] |

[a]Critical illness neuropathy [b]Acute tubular necrosis [C]Critical illness myopathy [d]Intracranial hemorrhage [e]Chronic obstructive pulmonary disease [f]combined critical illness neuropathy and myopathy (neuromyopathic syndrome) [g]Lower motor neuron [h]Upper motor neuron [I]Acute motor axonal neuropathy [J]Acute motor and sensory axonal neuropathy

**Table 1.** Characteristics of ill patients with profound weakness, who were referred for electrodiagnosis

Needle EMG of the diaphragm muscle is performed in cases with phrenic nerve involvement accompanying CIN as well as CIM. For this purpose, needle is inserted between the two Anterior Axillary and Medial clavicular lines, through 7$^{th}$ or 8$^{th}$ intercostal spaces, exactly over the rib. Neurogenic or myogenic patterns with or without fib/psw could be detected in inspiration phase of respiration [6].

Phrenic nerve EDX was requested for 4 of 14 patients in the present study. In two patients diagnosed with CIN and mixed neuromyopathic syndrome, there was no phrenic nerve involvement. In one patient secondary to AMAN, phrenic neuropathy was detected as bilateral asymmetric low amplitude CMAPs associated with neurogenic pattern in the diaphragm muscle and in one patient secondary to CIM, phrenic nerve involvement was revealed as bilateral absent CMAPs along with fib/psw and myogenic pattern in diaphragm muscle.

It should however be borne in mind that phrenic nerve EDX is mostly helpful whenever bilateral normal or unilateral abnormal responses are detected. In other words, if responses would be absent bilaterally it is difficult to distinguish from technical reasons [2].

**Treatment:** There is no specific treatment for CIN and supportive measures should be taken to avoid multi organ failure occurrence.

## 5. Critical Illness Myopathy (CIM)

The most common muscular disorder leading to weakness in ICU is critical illness myopathy. CIM is also known as acute quadriplegic myopathy, thick filament myopathy and ICU myopathy [1,2].

CIM is mostly seen concomitant to the administration of intravenous steroids and NMBAs; this complication is frequent in patients with asthma, COPD and administration of high-dose intravenous methyl-prednisolone [1].

Occurrence of one case of CIM and one case of mixed CIM/CIN in our patients' series with the history of hospitalization due to COPD exacerbation or corpulmonale confirms this fact (Table 1). This disorder however could also be seen in critically ill patients with sepsis or multiorgan failure without history of receiving corticosteroids or NMBAs. Prolonged mechanical ventilation per se even with absence of mentioned medications usage could cause CIM as well. In some cases, CIM is associated with increase in serum CPK levels (up to 10 times the upper limit of normal) [1]. High mortality rates with CIM; even a rate of 30% have been reported [4]. Of course, it should be noticed that the mortality cause has mostly been due to the sepsis or multiorgan failure rather than the myopathy itself. In present study, one case with pure CIM and one case with CIN were expired (Table 1). Survived and treated patients would acquire ambulation ability within the following 3-4 months [1].

From the histopathologic aspect, type II muscle fiber atrophy is observed more frequently than type I. In muscle biopsy, specific signs of myosin loss is often detected which solely could not explain the inexcitability of the muscle membrane that occurs with this myopathy.

Therefore, the following three factors contributing to reduction in muscle membrane excitability are introduced [7]:

1. Partial depolarization of the resting membrane potential,
2. Reduced membrane resistance,
3. Decreased sodium currents

Furthermore, released cytokines throughout sepsis could be associated with a catabolic state in muscles and results in breakdown of structural proteins [1,7].

## 6. Electrophysiologic features in CIM

Nerve conduction studies demonstrate diminished amplitudes of CMAPs with normal distal latencies and conduction velocities. In contrast, SNAPs are normal or mildly reduced (greater than 80% of lower limit of normal) [1]. Repetitive stimulation test (RST) is usually normal, but in some studies decreasing response after high rate and low rate RST have also been reported [8].

Electromyography frequently demonstrates prominent fibrillation potentials and positive sharp waves (fib/psw), which is rarely accompanied by myotoinc discharges. Short duration, small –amplitude and polyphasic MUAPs that recruit early are evident. In severe cases, it may be difficult to recruit and activate any MUAPs [1]. Of course, this process is reversed and small MUAPs will be appeared again during the recovery period.

### 6.1. Direct muscle stimulation technique

Direct muscle stimulation technique is utilized for differentiation CIM from critical illness neuropathy. This method has been reported by Rich and colleagues for first time [7, 9]. In fact, direct muscle stimulation bypasses distal motor nerve and neuromuscular junction area. This technique is performed by placing a monopolar needle stimulating electrode as cathode in the distal third of muscle using 0.1 msec stimulus duration with gradually increasing current from 10 to 100 mA until a clear twitch is seen. A subdermal needle electrode as active recording electrode is placed 1-3 cm from the stimulation electrode. The stimulation intensity is increased until a maximal response or direct muscle action potential (dm CMAP) is obtained. Next, using the same recording montage, nerve to the muscle is stimulated in the usual manner to obtain a nerve- evoked compound muscle action potential (ne CMAP) [2]. As a result muscle membrane should retain its excitability, direct muscle stimulation CMAP (dm CMAP) should be near normal despite a low or absent nerve stimulation evoked CMAP (ne CMAP). In contrast, if the muscle membrane excitability is reduced, both the ne CMAP and dm CMAP should be very low [1]. Therefore, in CIM as well as normal people, the ne CMAP/ dm CMAP ratio is close to one (1:1), because both amplitudes is proportionally reduced or normal, respectively. In CIN or neuromuscular junction disorder, the ratio is much lower and approaches zero because of disproportionally lower ne CMAP compared with the dm CMAP.

In conclusion, absent or low amplitude of dm CMAP with ne CMAP/ dm CMAP greater than 0.9 is demonstrated in majority of patients with CIM, While ne CMAP/ dm CMAP ratio is 0.5 or less in patients with severe CIN [1].

### 6.2. Treatment

There is no medical therapy other than supportive care and treating underlying systemic abnormalities (e.g., antibiotics in sepsis). If patients are still receiving high doses of corticosteroids or non- depolarizing neuromuscular blockers, the medications should be stopped.

## 7. Critical illness neuropathy in combination with myopathy (Neuromyopathic syndrome)

Patients occasionally present with combination of CIN and CIM symptoms, which make it complicated to distinguish or detect from each other [1].This condition is named as Neuromyopathic Syndrome.

In our patients' series, Neuromyopathic Syndrome was observed in 4 from 14 patients, two of whom had a combination of CIN and CIM. Third case admitted with chronic severe motor and sensory neuropathy symptoms; later presence of myogenic pattern in needle EMG revealed additional CIM. Forth patient suffered from FUO (Fever unknown origin) and demonstrated CIM which had been superimposed on previously diagnosed AMAN. (Table1). One explanation is partly related to this fact, that preexisting neuropathic aspects in these patients were completed parallel to disease progression and subsequently myogenic process and thick filament myopathy initiated following intubation and administration of NMBAs and corticosteroids. We categorized these cases in "Neuromyopathic Syndrome" or "combination of critical illness neuropathy and myopathy" group.

### 7.1. Electrophysiologic features in combined CIN/CIM

NCS shows CMAPs and SNAPs both are low amplitude or unobtainable. NCVs are reduced but within axonal range (greater than 60-70% of lower limit of normal). Despite of these neuropathic features, myogenic process with low amplitude, short duration and polyphasic MUAPs are mostly seen, which is occasionally associated with patchy neurogenic changes in needle electromyography examination.

Table 2 illustrates the electrodiagnostic changes in differential diagnosis among critically ill patients.

| | Low amplitude or absent SNAP | Low amplitude or absent CMAP | Reduced NCV > 60-70% of LLN[a] | fib/psw[b] | Myogenic Pattern | Neurogenic Pattern |
|---|---|---|---|---|---|---|
| CIN[c] | ++ | ++ | - | ++ | - | ++ |
| CIM[d] | - | ++ | - | +++ | ++ | - |
| GBS[e] | +/- | +/- | ++ | - | - | + |
| AMAN[f] | - | + | - | ++ | - | ++ |
| AMSAN[g] | + | + | - | + | - | + |
| CIN/CIM[h] | + | + | - | ++ | + | +/- |

[a]Lower Limit of Normal, [b]Fibrillation Potentials, [c]Critical Illness Neuropathy, [d]Critical Illness Myopathy, [e]Gullian Barre Syndrome, [f]Acute Motor Axonal Neuropathy, [g]Acute Motor and Sensory Axonal Neuropathy, [h]combination of CIN and CIM (Neuromyopathic syndrome)

**Table 2.** Electrodiagnostic changes in various neuromuscular disorders among critically ill patients

## 8. Prolonged Neuromuscular Junction Blockage:

Neuromuscular junction block (NMJ block) occurs primarily in diseases like Myastenia gravis and Lambert-Eaton myastenic syndrome without simultaneous myopathy or neuropathy. However, this complication is frequently observed in association with CIN or CIM in critically ill patients who secondarily affected by neuromuscular disorders.

The definite diagnosis is achieved by performing RST or RNS (Repetitive Nerve Stimulation Test) and appearance of decreasing responses and fatigue following repetitive stimulation of low rates at 2-3 Hz in Myastenia gravis or NMJ block in combination with CIM. In contrast, increment responses and facilitation are observed following stimulation of high rates at 25-50 Hz in Lambert-Eaton syndrome [10].

It should be mentioned that pure NMJ block are rarely seen in these patients. In the present study, RST was not performed to confirm the simultaneous NMJ block for referred patients, who were critically ill and poorly cooperative with definite diagnosis in each category of CIN, CIM, AMAN, etc., because of this fact that RST tests are time consuming, painful and somewhat unnecessary, since it does not add extra benefit concerning the final therapeutic process as well as prognosis in this spectrum of patients.

In the previous sections, approaches to critically ill patients suspected of having neuropathy or myopathy were reviewed, now we turn our focus to the other neuropathies ,which are in the differential diagnostic list of profound weakness in the inpatient or ICU setting. These disorders are often amenable to treat, so correct diagnosis is important.

## 9. Acute inflammatory demylinating polyradiculoneuropathy (AIDP)

The most well known acute neuropathy that results in marked weakness and respiratory compromise is Guillain-Barre syndrome (GBS) [2]. GBS is an acquired motor and sensory polyradiculneuopathy that is usually demylinating.

### 9.1. Electrophysiologic features in GBS

Demylinating is prescribed with motor nerve conduction velocity less than 60-70% of LLN (lower limit of normal),prolonged distal motor latencies and F-waves greater than 25-50% of ULN( upper limit of normal), absent F-waves and presence of conduction block or temporal dispersion in one or more motor nerves in electrodiagnostic studies. These criteria have been defined and reported by Cornblath et al, and are used as research criteria for diagnosis of GBS since 1990 [11,12].

In our patients' series, there was no case of GBS and as previously mentioned most of them were hospitalized due to primary non-neurologic medical reasons and CIN or CIM was added later. Other cases that were presented with weakness in upper and lower extremities with or without other medical problems were included in axonal variants of GBS, which is discussed as follows.

## 10. Acute motor and sensory axonal neuropathy (AMSAN)

Feasby and colleagues initially reported this axonal variant of GBS in 1986 [13]. Clinical and electrodiagnostic features in AMSAN are indistinguishable from those with AIDP initially [5]. Patients with AMSAN refer with a rapidly progressive and generalized weakness which progresses within days unlike the AIDP which progresses within weeks. Ophthalmoparesia, swallowing disorders, and facial muscles weakness are prominent in these patients. Other accompanying symptoms include complete areflexia, sensory loss and autonomic disorders such as arrhythmia. Most of these patients would require ventilator and their prognosis are often poorer compared with AIDP patients.

### 10.1. Electrophysiologic features in AMSAN

NCS reveal markedly diminished amplitudes or absent CMAPs. SNAPs are also profoundly low amplitude or absent. But distal latencies of CMAPs and NCVs, when obtainable, should be normal or only mildly affected [5] .In other words, this abnormality would be within axonal range(greater than 60-70% of LLN). Neurogenic pattern with large MUAPs with or without denervation potentials are seen in needle EMG exam (Table 2).

In the present study, there was one case with AMSAN had started with above-mentioned clinical picture followed by COPD exacerbation and diagnosis was confirmed by EDX criteria.

### 10.2. Treatment

Because it is difficult to distinguish AIDP from AMSAN clinically or electrophysiologically, at least initially, treatment with plasma exchange or IVIG is warranted [5].

## 11. Acute Motor Axonal Neuropathy (AMAN)

In northern china, AMAN is the most common variant of GBS [14].Clinical manifestation is similar to that of AMSAN and GBS, however distal muscles are affected more severely than proximal muscles. Respiratory failure and mechanical ventilation requirement is observed in one third of the patients. Unlike AMSAN and GBS no sensory sings are noted. Furthermore, Anti-GM1 antibody for Compilobacter jejuni is more frequently detected in patients with AMAN especially in Children [15].

### 11.1. Electrophysiologic features in AMAN

Low amplitude or absent CMAPs with normal SNAPs and mildly reduced NCVs, are the characteristic features of nerve conduction studies in AMAN. Other EDx evidences are similar to AMSAN as above noted.

In our patients' series, there were two cases with AMAN from whom one case was associated with phrenic nerve involvement and diaphragm muscle paralysis with respiratory disturbances. There was also a case without respiratory involvement with an appropriate response to IVIG (Table 1).

### 11.2. Treatment

It is suggested to treat AMAN patients with IVIG 2mg/kg over 5 days or plasma exchange as an alternative. One of large studies reported no significant difference in outcome regardless of therapy (IVIG,PE,..) between AIDP and AMAN among 300 patients[15].

**In conclusion**, CIN and CIM have no cure, so in this conditions, underlying disease and drugs dose should be treated and adjusted, respectively; despite of this management, muscle power weakness lasts several months to recover. AIDP, AMAN and AMSAN, however, are curable and therefore distinguish them together is important.

## Author details

Fariba Eslamian and Mohammad Rahbar
*Tabriz University of Medical Sciences, Physical medicine & Rehabilitation Research Center, Tabriz, Iran*

## 12. References

[1] Dumitru D, Amato AA (2002) Acquired myopathies. In: Dumitru D, Amato AA, Zwarts MJ, editors. Electrodiagnostic medicine. 2nd ed. Philadelphia, PA: Hanley & Belfus Inc; pp. 1402-1404.

[2] Preston DC, Shapiro BE (2005) Approach to Electrodiagnostic Studies in the Intensive Care Unit. In: Preston DC, Shapiro BE, eds. Electromyography and Neuromuscular disorders. 2nd ed. Philadelphia, Elsevier. pp.615-625

[3] Op de Coul AAW, Lambregts PC, Koeman J,et al (1985) Neuromuscular complications in patients given Pavulon during artificial ventilation. Clin Neurol Neurosurg . 87:17-20.

[4] Lacomis D, Petrella JT, Giuliani MJ (1998) Causes of neuromuscular weakness in the intensive care unit: a study of ninety-two patients. Muscle Nerve. 21(5):610-7

[5] Dumitru D, Amato AA (2002) Acquired neuropathies In: Dumitru D, Amato AA, Zwarts MJ, editors. Electrodiagnostic medicine. 2nd ed. Philadelphia, PA: Hanley & Belfus Inc; pp.937-989.

[6] Dumitru D, Zwarts MJ (2002) Focal cranial neuropathies. In: Dumitru D, Amato AA, Zwarts MJ, editors. Electrodiagnostic medicine. 2nd ed. Philadelphia, PA: Hanley & Belfus Inc; pp.688-690.

[7] Rich MM, Teener JW, Raps EC, Schotland DL, Bird SJ (1996) Muscle is electrically unexcitable in acute quadriplegic myopathy. Neurology. 46(3):731-6

[8] Road J, Mackie G, Jiang TX, Stewart H, Eisen A (1997) Reversible paralysis with status asthmaticus, steroids, and pancuronium: clinical electrophysiological correlates. Muscle Nerve. 20(12):1587-90

[9] Rich MM, Bird SJ, Raps EC, McCluskey LF, Teener JW (1997) Direct muscle stimulation in acute quadriplegic myopathy. Muscle Nerve. 20(6):665-673.
[10] Dumitru D, Amato AA (2002) Neuromuscular junction disorders. In: Dumitru D, Amato AA, Zwarts MJ, eds. Electrodiagnostic medicine. 2nd ed. Philadelphia, PA: Hanley & Belfus Inc. pp.1148-1177.
[11] Cornblath DR, Asbury AK, Albers JW (1991) Research criteria for diagnosis of chronic inflammatory demyelinating polyneuropathy (CIDP). Neurology. 41:617-618.
[12] Cornblath DR, Mellits ED, Griffin JW, McKhann GM, Albers JW, Miller RG, Feasby TE, Quaskey SA (1988) Motor conduction studies in Guillain-Barré syndrome: description and prognostic value. Ann Neurol. 23(4):354-359.
[13] Feasby TE, Gilbert JJ, Brown WF, Bolton CF, Hahn AF, Koopman WF, Zochodne DW (1986) An acute axonal form of Guillain-Barré polyneuropathy. Brain. 109 (Pt 6):1115-1126.
[14] McKhann GM, Cornblath DR, Ho T, Li CY, Bai AY, Wu HS, Yei QF, Zhang WC, Zhaori 11 Z, Jiang Z, et al. (1991) Clinical and electrophysiological aspects of acute paralytic disease of children and young adults in northern China. Lancet. 7; 338(8767):593-597.
[15] Hadden RD, Cornblath DR, Hughes RA, Zielasek J, Hartung HP, Toyka KV, Swan AV (1998) Electrophysiological classification of Guillain-Barré syndrome: clinical associations and outcome. Plasma Exchange/Sandoglobulin Guillain-Barré Syndrome Trial Group. Ann Neurol. 44(5):780-788.

Chapter 6

# Pacemaker Neurons and Neuronal Networks in Health and Disease

Fernando Peña-Ortega

Additional information is available at the end of the chapter

http://dx.doi.org/10.5772/50264

## 1. Introduction

Neural network activity provides the operational basis for diverse neural circuits to determine temporal windows during which multiple, coherent neuronal assemblies engaged in the generation of specific behaviors can be recruited [1-3]. Neural network activity emerges from the combination of intrinsic neural properties and the synaptic interactions among them [1-5]. However, the relative contributions of intrinsic and synaptic properties to circuit activity are diverse and change, depending on the state of the network, mainly through the action of neuromodulators [6]. On top of this diversity, the intrinsic properties of neurons are also heterogeneous, ranging from silent "linear" neurons (also called followers or non-pacemakers; Fig 1 bottom trace) to "non-linear" intrinsic bursters (also called pacemakers; Fig. 1 upper trace) [7]. The presence of pacemaker neurons and their pivotal role in network activity generation is an accepted fact for invertebrate networks [8]. In the case of mammalian circuits, accumulating evidence supports the presence and participation of these pacemakers in generating network rhythmic activity by several circuits throughout the brain in normal and abnormal conditions [1,4,5, 9-11]. In mammalian networks, bursting has been related to neural network generation [1], induction of synaptic plasticity, [12] as well as to the transition of abnormal neural network states [13,14]. Here, I will review just some examples of neural networks that contain pacemaker neurons, the main ionic mechanisms involved in their bursting generation, and the participation of these pacemakers in generating neural network function under normal and pathological conditions.

For the purpose of this chapter, pacemakers are defined as neurons that can generate oscillatory bursts of action potentials independently of the network, i.e. in the absence of any synaptic input [Fig. 1; upper trace] [1,9]. They do so because they have a mixture of ionic conductances that allow them to produce rhythmic excursions of the membrane potential on top of which barrages of action potentials are generated [3; 11; Fig. 1; upper trace]. In networks that contain them, pacemaker neurons may act as true pacemakers or as resonators that respond preferentially to specific firing frequencies [1,9]. Non-pacemaker neurons change their firing rate gradually in almost strict correspondence to their synaptic input [1]. In contrast, the nonlinearity of bursting activity enables pacemaker neurons to modulate more abruptly their firing [1]. Moreover, bursting neurons amplify synaptic input and transmit their information more reliably through synaptic contacts [15-17]. As a consequence of these properties, pacemaker neurons can facilitate the onset of excitatory states or synchronize neuronal ensembles involved in diverse functional roles, such as movement control, sleep-wakefulness cycling, perception, attention, etc. [1,9]. The ability of these neurons to generate bursts of action potentials lies in voltage-sensitive ion fluxes, which act in specific voltage- and time-windows and whose activity is regulated by the metabolic state of the neurons, by neuromodulators, and by activity-dependent mechanisms [1, 18-20]. Next, I will describe some examples of mammalian neural networks containing pacemaker neurons.

One of the more popular examples of a mammalian pacemaker neuron is, perhaps, the reticular thalamic neuron (RTN) [22,23]. RTNs are able to generate bursts of action potentials depending on two major inward currents: the low-threshold (T-type) Ca2+ channels [22,23] and the hyperpolarization-activated and cyclic nucleotide-gated nonselective cation channel (HCN) [24]. Interestingly, these neurons can switch from the "bursting mode" to a "tonic mode" depending on their membrane potential [25,26]. The transitions between firing modes are determined by the action of several neuromodulators as well as by GABAergic phasic inhibition [25,26]. It has been proposed that the "bursting mode" of these RTNs dominates the generation of slow-wave activity during non-REM sleep, whereas the transition to the tonic firing mode is related to the generation of faster rhythms produced during wakefulness [25,26]. Therefore, it has been proposed that pacemaker RTN neurons are key elements of the cortico-thalamic neural network that gates the transitions among different states of consciousness [i.e. sleep/awakening] [22,23]. From a clinical point of view, it has been reported that an increase during wakefulness of the bursting mode of RTN neurons is related to the generation of absence seizures [27,28]. Accordingly, absence seizures are successfully treated with T-type Ca2+ channel blockers such as ethosuximide, which reduces the bursting mode of RTNs [28,29].

Intrinsic bursting neurons have been identified in the neocortex [30-34]. These pacemakers correspond to a subgroup of pyramidal neurons and to a subset of Martinotti-interneuron cells [30-33]. As expected, pacemaker pyramidal cells are functionally and anatomical different from regular spiking (RS) pyramidal neurons. For example, intrinsic bursters have specific morphological features that differentiate them from the typical pyramidal RS neurons [31]. Intrinsic bursters are larger than RS neurons; they have a triangular soma rather than the more rounded soma of RS pyramidal neurons and a more complex dendritic tree [31]. Regarding their projection, intrinsic bursters send collaterals that are limited to layers 5/6, whereas axonal collaterals from RS pyramidal neurons are more pronounced in

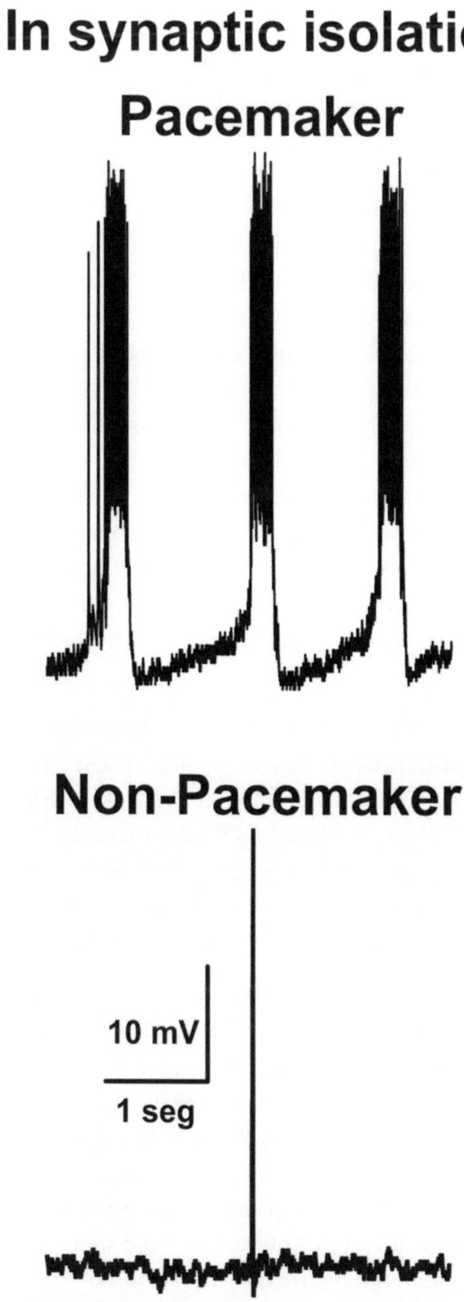


**Figure 1. Identification of pacemaker and non-pacemaker neurons.** Recordings from two neurons in the preBötzinger Complex are shown in conditions where fast synaptic transmission has been blocked using a cocktail of glutamate, GABA, and glycine receptor antagonists (synaptic isolation). Whereas both neurons were originally identified as rhythmic inspiratory neurons, in synaptic isolation pacemakers can be identified by their ability to continue the generation of oscillatory bursts of action potentials independently of the network. In contrast, non-pacemaker neurons become either silent or fire tonically in a non-rhythmic fashion.

the supragranular layers [31, 34, 35]. Moreover, the intracortical circuits for intrinsic bursters are different from those of RS neurons [35]. For instance, intrinsic bursters receive intracolumnar excitatory innervations from all layers, whereas RS neurons receive intracolumnar inhibitory and excitatory inputs from layers 2/3 and 5 [35]. Finally, the extracortical projections of these two types of pyramidal cells differ; for instance, intrinsic bursters project to the thalamus, pons, and colliculus while RS neurons project to cortical and striatal targets [36,37]. Cortical pacemakers have been hypothesized to play a major role in the generation of spontaneous activity [4, 33]. For instance, Cunningham et al. [4] have described a group of intrinsic pacemakers that produce bursts of action potentials in the gamma range, relying on the persistent sodium current (INap), and that their blockade abolishes gamma generation in the auditory cortex. Similarly, other types of intrinsic bursters that also rely on the INap, but that fire their bursts at lower frequencies, have been implicated in the generation of population activity in the somatosensory cortex [38,39]. Based on this and other evidence, it has been proposed that the cortex may act as a central pattern generator [2]. From a pathological point of view, cortical pacemaker neurons play a role in the generation of epileptic network activity [13; 14]. For example, we have found that human cortical epileptic foci have an increased number of cells with INap-dependent pacemaker properties [13,14], which may explain why reducing the INap has an antiepileptic effect [40-42].

Similarly to gamma rhythm, pacemakers involved in theta rhythm generation have been identified in the septohippocampal network [10,43]. These putative theta pacemaker neurons are GABAergic cells that are localized in the medial septum and express parvalbumin and the HCN [44-46]. Interestingly, alterations in the activity of these theta pacemaker neurons might be involved in the pathophysiology of Alzheimer disease (AD), which progresses with a reduction in evoked-theta oscillations [47]. Accordingly, application of the AD-related amyloid-beta peptide reduces the activity of theta-pacemaker neurons and reduces theta rhythm in rats [43, 48-50].

Pacemaker neurons have been reported in the hypothalamic arcuate nucleus, which is responsible for the control of the satiety-hunger cycle [51]. These neurons, which contain neuropeptide Y [NPY], are conditional pacemakers that are activated by orexigens (ghrelin and orexin) and inhibited by the anorexigens (leptin) [51]. The busting properties of these neurons do not depend on the INap, because their membrane potential oscillations persist in the presence of tetrodotoxin, but are inhibited by blocking the T-type calcium channel [51]. Since these arcuate pacemakers can contribute to balanced food consumption, an alteration in their activity can be associated with eating disorders and obesity [52-54].

Subthalamic neurons can exhibit bursting properties, depending on the state of the network. As RTNs, subthalamic pacemakers can shift from a regular, single-spike mode to a burst-firing mode depending on their depolarization level [55,56]. The bursting mode relies on the L-type and the T-type Ca2+ channels, and it is insensitive to tetrodotoxin [55,57]. The subthalamic nucleus is composed of glutamatergic neurons, whose normal transition between tonic and bursting modes controls the circuitry of the basal ganglia by modulating the activity of the two principal output structures of the network: the internal pallidal segment and the substantia nigra pars reticulata [58, 55, 56]. Interestingly, pacemaker activity of subthalamic neurons has been associated with Parkinson's disease [59]. For instance, an increase in subthalamic burst firing has been found in animal models of parkinsonism [60,61] and in parkinsonian patients [62,63]. Also noteworthy is that high-frequency stimulation of the subthalamic nucleus, which reduces subthalamic busrstiness [62,64], produces a reduction in motor impairments associated with parkinsonism and is currently used in the treatment of parkinsonian patients [63,65]. Moreover, modulation of the T-type calcium channel in subthalamic busrters also reduces parkinsonisms [66].

Pacemaker neurons have also been identified in the spinal cord, where they seem to play a major role in its central pattern generators [67-69]. For instance, in the central pattern generator for locomotion, some interneurons exhibit intrinsic bursting activity [67-69] that relies on the INap [67-69]. This mechanism is essential for the activity of the locomotion central pattern generator, since blockade of INap abolishes bursting activity and fictive locomotion [67-69]. Also in the spinal cord, it was recently reported that an increase in pacemaker activity is observed in the dorsal horn of animals that suffer from chronic pain [70]. These intrinsic bursters exhibit an increase in the density of the INap and the HCN [70], which may offer therapeutic targets to treat chronic pain [71,72]. In fact, several blockers of the INap have shown very promising effects against acute and chronic pain [73-75]. Finally, I will review the role of pacemaker neurons in the activity of a vital network: the preBötzinger Complex (preBötC).

## 2. Role of pacemakers can be state-dependent: An example of the inspiratory rhythm generator

Respiratory rhythm commands are generated by two, interacting oscillators, one controlling inspiration (preBötC) and other, located in the parafacial respiratory group (pFRG), possibly controlling active expiration [76-79]. Neurons with pacemaker properties have been identified in the preBötC [5,80,81; Fig. 1]. However, a rather complex picture has emerged regarding their intrinsic properties. PreBötC pacemakers have been found to show considerable variability in the range of interburst and intraburst frequencies, the amplitude of the plateau potential underlying bursting firing, and the voltage trajectory of this plateau [5, 80-86]. A biophysical and pharmacological characterization of their intrinsic properties have shown us that preBötC pacemakers can be grouped into two major groups: those that rely on the INap and those that rely on a Ca2+-activated non-specific cationic current [ICAN] [5, 82, 84, 86]. Interestingly, the participation of these pacemakers in respiratory rhythm generation is state dependent. We found that blocking either the pacemakers that rely on the INap or the pacemakers that rely on the ICAN is not sufficient to abolish respiratory rhythm generation by the preBötC [5, 87]. However, when both of the two pacemaker populations are blocked, the preBötC ceases the generation of its rhythmic activity [5], and the animals die [87]. This evidence suggests that breathing generation relies on the activity of two distinct pacemaker neurons [5,87]. However, this is not the case when the preBötC is challenged with hypoxic conditions. During hypoxia, the respiratory network is reconfigured and generates a "last-resort" respiratory rhythm called gasping [79]. Under these conditions the pacemaker neurons relying on the ICAN cease to fire, and the respiratory network relies only on the INap-dependent pacemaker neuron, whose blockade abolishes gasping generation [5,87]. These findings may have clinical relevance since gasping is an important autoresuscitation mechanism that seems to fail in victims of sudden infant death syndrome [SIDS, 88,89]. SIDS victims breathe normally during normoxia, when the respiratory rhythm can be generated by either of the two types of pacemaker, but they do not gasp efficiently in hypoxia [88,89], when the respiratory network relies exclusively on one type of pacemaker neuron.

## 3. Conclusion

In conclusion, pacemaker neurons are important components of several mammalian neural networks. The presence of pacemaker neurons allows these networks to produce different types of network activities, both in normal and in pathological conditions. Moreover, the contribution of pacemaker neurons to neural network dynamics is not fixed but depends on the action of neuromodulators or the state of the network. I believe that pacemaker neurons provide neural networks with the ability to coordinate population activity and to adjust it in response to several physiological demands. Unfortunately, changes in pacemaker activity can also lead to pathological states associated with several neurological diseases. The study of pacemaker properties, which is a very interesting topic itself, may also identify molecular targets to correct abnormal network activity.

## Author details

Fernando Peña-Ortega
*Instituto de Neurobiología, UNAM, México*

## Acknowledgement

I would like to thank Dorothy Pless for reviewing the English version of this paper. The research in my lab has been sponsored by grants from DGAPA IB200212, CONACyT 151261, and from the Alzheimer's Association NIRG-11-205443.

## 4. References

[1] Ramirez JM, Tryba AK, Peña F (2004) Pacemaker neurons and neuronal networks: an integrative view. Curr. Opin. Neurobiol. 14:665-674.

[2] Yuste R, MacLean JN, Smith J, Lansner A (2005) The cortex as a central pattern generator. Nat. Rev. Neurosci. 6:477-483.

[3] Peña-Ortega F (2011) Possible role or respiratory pacemaker neurons in the generation of different breathing patterns. En: Pacemakers, Theory and Applications. Transworld Research Network., pp. Intech Open Acces Publisher

[4] Cunningham MO, Whittington MA, Bibbig A, Roopun A, LeBeau FE, Vogt A, Monyer H, Buhl EH, Traub RD (2004) A role for fast rhythmic bursting neurons in cortical gamma oscillations in vitro. Proc. Natl. Acad. Sci. U. S. A. 101:7152-7157.

[5] Peña F, Parkis MA, Tryba AK, Ramirez JM (2004) Differential contribution of pacemaker properties to the generation of respiratory rhythms during normoxia and hypoxia. Neuron. 43:105-117.

[6] Doi A, Ramirez JM (2010) State-dependent interactions between excitatory neuromodulators in the neuronal control of breathing. J. Neurosci. 30:8251-8262.

[7] Butera RJ Jr, Rinzel J, Smith JC (1999) Models of respiratory rhythm generation in the pre-Bötzinger complex. I. Bursting pacemaker neurons. J. Neurophysiol. 82:382-397.

[8] Marder E, Manor Y, Nadim F, Bartos M, Nusbaum MP (1998) Frequency control of a slow oscillatory network by a fast rhythmic input: pyloric to gastric mill interactions in the crab stomatogastric nervous system. Ann. N. Y. Acad. Sci. 860:226-238.

[9] Llinás RR (1988) The intrinsic electrophysiological properties of mammalian neurons: insights into central nervous system function. Science. 242:1654-1664.

[10] Wang XJ (2002) Pacemaker neurons for the theta rhythm and their synchronization in the septohippocampal reciprocal loop. J. Neurophysiol. 87:889-900.

[11] Peña F. Contribution of pacemaker neurons to respiratory rhythms generation in vitro. Adv. Exp. Med. Biol. 2008 605:114-118.

[12] Pike FG, Meredith RM, Olding AW, Paulsen O (1999) Rapid report: postsynaptic bursting is essential for 'Hebbian' induction of associative long-term potentiation at excitatory synapses in rat hippocampus. J. Physiol. 518:571-576.

[13] Marcuccilli CJ, Tryba AK, van Drongelen W, Koch H, Viemari JC, Peña-Ortega F, Doren EL, Pytel P, Chevalier M, Mrejeru A, Kohrman MH, Lasky RE, Lew SM, Frim DM, Ramirez JM (2010) Neuronal bursting properties in focal and parafocal regions in pediatric neocortical epilepsy stratified by histology. J. Clin. Neurophysiol. 27:387-397.

[14] Tryba AK, Kaczorowski CC, Ben-Mabrouk F, Elsen FP, Lew SM, Marcuccilli CJ (2011) Rhythmic intrinsic bursting neurons in human neocortex obtained from pediatric patients with epilepsy. Eur. J. Neurosci. 34:31-44.

[15] Snider RK, Kabara JF, Roig BR, Bonds AB (1998) Burst firing and modulation of functional connectivity in cat striate cortex. J. Neurophysiol. 80:730-744.

[16] Csicsvari J, Hirase H, Czurko A, Buzsáki G (1998) Reliability and state dependence of pyramidal cell-interneuron synapses in the hippocampus: an ensemble approach in the behaving rat. Neuron. 21:179-189.

[17] Williams SR, Stuart GJ (1999) Mechanisms and consequences of action potential burst firing in rat neocortical pyramidal neurons. J. Physiol. 521:467-482.

[18] Zhang W, Linden DJ (2003) The other side of the engram: experience-driven changes in neuronal intrinsic excitability. Nat. Rev. Neurosci. 4:885-900.

[19] Harris-Warrick RM (2002) Voltage-sensitive ion channels in rhythmic motor systems. Curr. Opin. Neurobiol. 12:646-651.

[20] Harris-Warrick RM (2011) Neuromodulation and flexibility in Central Pattern Generator networks. Curr. Opin. Neurobiol. 21:685-692.

[21] Williams SR, Stuart GJ (1999) Mechanisms and consequences of action potential burst firing in rat neocortical pyramidal neurons. J. Physiol. 521:467-482.

[22] Zhang L, Renaud LP, Kolaj M (2009) Properties of a T-type Ca2+channel-activated slow afterhyperpolarization in thalamic paraventricular nucleus and other thalamic midline neurons. J. Neurophysiol. 101:2741-2750.

[23] Astori S, Wimmer RD, Prosser HM, Corti C, Corsi M, Liaudet N, Volterra A, Franken P, Adelman JP, Lüthi A (2011) The Ca(V)3.3 calcium channel is the major sleep spindle pacemaker in thalamus. Proc. Natl. Acad. Sci. U. S. A. 108:13823-8.

[24] Lüthi A, Bal T, McCormick DA (1998) Periodicity of thalamic spindle waves is abolished by ZD7288,a blocker of Ih. J. Neurophysiol. 79:3284-3289.

[25] Leresche N, Jassik-Gerschenfeld D, Haby M, Soltesz I, Crunelli V (1990) Pacemaker-like and other types of spontaneous membrane potential oscillations of thalamocortical cells. Neurosci. Lett. 113:72-77.

[26] McCormick DA, Williamson A (1991) Modulation of neuronal firing mode in cat and guinea pig LGNd by histamine: possible cellular mechanisms of histaminergic control of arousal. J. Neurosci. 11:3188-3199.

[27] Zhang Y, Vilaythong AP, Yoshor D, Noebels JL (2004) Elevated thalamic low-voltage-activated currents precede the onset of absence epilepsy in the SNAP25-deficient mouse mutant coloboma. J. Neurosci. 24:5239-5248.

[28] Broicher T, Seidenbecher T, Meuth P, Munsch T, Meuth SG, Kanyshkova T, Pape HC, Budde T (2007) T-current related effects of antiepileptic drugs and a Ca2+ channel antagonist on thalamic relay and local circuit interneurons in a rat model of absence epilepsy. Neuropharmacology. 53:431-446.

[29] Tringham E, Powell KL, Cain SM, Kuplast K, Mezeyova J, Weerapura M, Eduljee C, Jiang X, Smith P, Morrison JL, Jones NC, Braine E, Rind G, Fee-Maki M, Parker D, Pajouhesh H, Parmar M, O'Brien TJ, Snutch TP (2012) T-type calcium channel blockers that attenuate thalamic burst firing and suppress absence seizures. Sci. Transl. Med. 4:121ra19.

[30] Agmon A, Connors BW (1992) Correlation between intrinsic firing patterns and thalamocortical synaptic responses of neurons in mouse barrel cortex. J. Neurosci. 12:319-329.

[31] Chagnac-Amitai Y, Luhmann HJ, Prince DA (1990) Burst generating and regular spiking layer 5 pyramidal neurons of rat neocortex have different morphological features. J. Comp. Neurol. 296:598-613.

[32] Zhu JJ, Connors BW (1999) Intrinsic firing patterns and whisker-evoked synaptic responses of neurons in the rat barrel cortex. J. Neurophysiol. 81:1171-1183.

[33] Le Bon-Jego M, Yuste R (2007) Persistently active, pacemaker-like neurons in neocortex. Front. Neurosci. 1:123-129.

[34] Jacob V, Petreanu L, Wright N, Svoboda K, Fox K (2012) Regular spiking and intrinsic bursting pyramidal cells show orthogonal forms of experience-dependent plasticity in layer V of barrel cortex. Neuron. 73:391-404.

[35] Schubert D, Staiger JF, Cho N, Kötter R, Zilles K, Luhmann HJ (2001) Layer-specific intracolumnar and transcolumnar functional connectivity of layer V pyramidal cells in rat barrel cortex. J. Neurosci. 21:3580-3592.
[36] Gao WJ, Zheng ZH (2004) Target-specific differences in somatodendritic morphology of layer V pyramidal neurons in rat motor cortex. J. Comp. Neurol. 476:174-185.
[37] Le Bé JV, Silberberg G, Wang Y, Markram H (2007) Morphological, electrophysiological, and synaptic properties of corticocallosal pyramidal cells in the neonatal rat neocortex. Cereb. Cortex. 17:2204-2213.
[38] Mao BQ, Hamzei-Sichani F, Aronov D, Froemke RC, Yuste R (2001) Dynamics of spontaneous activity in neocortical slices. Neuron. 32:883-898.
[39] van Drongelen W, Koch H, Elsen FP, Lee HC, Mrejeru A, Doren E, Marcuccilli CJ, Hereld M, Stevens RL, Ramirez JM (2006) Role of persistent sodium current in bursting activity of mouse neocortical networks in vitro. J. Neurophysiol. 96:2564-2577.
[40] Taverna S, Mantegazza M, Franceschetti S, Avanzini G (1998) Valproate selectively reduces the persistent fraction of Na+ current in neocortical neurons. Epilepsy Res. 32:304-308.
[41] Taverna S, Sancini G, Mantegazza M, Franceschetti S, Avanzini G (1999) Inhibition of transient and persistent Na+ current fractions by the new anticonvulsant topiramate. J. Pharmacol. Exp. Ther. 288:960-8.
[42] Stafstrom CE (2007) Persistent sodium current and its role in epilepsy. Epilepsy Curr. 7:15-22.
[43] Villette V, Poindessous-Jazat F, Simon A, Léna C, Roullot E, Bellessort B, Epelbaum J, Dutar P, Stéphan A (2010) Decreased rhythmic GABAergic septal activity and memory-associated theta oscillations after hippocampal amyloid-beta pathology in the rat. J. Neurosci. 30:10991-11003.
[44] Simon AP, Poindessous-Jazat F, Dutar P, Epelbaum J, Bassant MH (2006) Firing properties of anatomically identified neurons in the medial septum of anesthetized and unanesthetized restrained rats. J. Neurosci. 26:9038-9046.
[45] Varga V, Hangya B, Kránitz K, Ludányi A, Zemankovics R, Katona I, Shigemoto R, Freund TF, Borhegyi Z (2008) The presence of pacemaker HCN channels identifies theta rhythmic GABAergic neurons in the medial septum. J. Physiol. 586:3893-915.
[46] Hangya B, Borhegyi Z, Szilágyi N, Freund TF, Varga V (2009) GABAergic neurons of the medial septum lead the hippocampal network during theta activity. J. Neurosci. 29:8094-8102.
[47] Cummins TD, Broughton M, Finnigan S (2008) Theta oscillations are affected by amnestic mild cognitive impairment and cognitive load. Int. J. Psychophysiol. 70:75-81.
[48] Peña F, Ordaz B, Balleza-Tapia H, Bernal-Pedraza R, Márquez-Ramos A, Carmona-Aparicio L, Giordano M (2010) Beta-amyloid protein (25-35) disrupts hippocampal network activity: role of Fyn-kinase. Hippocampus. 20:78-96.
[49] Colom LV, Castañeda MT, Bañuelos C, Puras G, García-Hernández A, Hernandez S, Mounsey S, Benavidez J, Lehker C (2010) Medial septal beta-amyloid 1-40 injections alter septo-hippocampal anatomy and function. Neurobiol. Aging. 31:46-57.

[50] Peña-Ortega f, Bernal-Pedraza R (2012) Amyloid beta slows down sensory-induced hippocampal oscillations, International Journal of Peptides, In press.
[51] van den Top M, Lee K, Whyment AD, Blanks AM, Spanswick D (2004) Orexigen-sensitive NPY/AgRP pacemaker neurons in the hypothalamic arcuate nucleus. Nat. Neurosci. 7:493-494.
[52] Davidowa H, Plagemann A (2000) Decreased inhibition by leptin of hypothalamic arcuate neurons in neonatally overfed young rats. Neuroreport. 11:2795-2798.
[53] Davidowa H, Plagemann A (2007) Insulin resistance of hypothalamic arcuate neurons in neonatally overfed rats. Neuroreport. 18:521-524.
[54] Mirshamsi S, Olsson M, Arnelo U, Kinsella JM, Permert J, Ashford ML (2007) BVT.3531 reduces body weight and activates K(ATP) channels in isolated arcuate neurons in rats. Regul. Pept. 141:19-24.
[55] Beurrier C, Congar P, Bioulac B, Hammond C (1999) Subthalamic nucleus neurons switch from single-spike activity to burst-firing mode. J. Neurosci. 19:599-609.
[56] Kass JI, Mintz IM (2006) Silent plateau potentials, rhythmic bursts, and pacemaker firing: three patterns of activity that coexist in quadristable subthalamic neurons. Proc. Natl. Acad. Sci. U. S. A. 103:183-188.
[57] Baufreton J, Garret M, Rivera A, de la Calle A, Gonon F, Dufy B, Bioulac B, Taupignon A (2003) D5 (not D1) dopamine receptors potentiate burst-firing in neurons of the subthalamic nucleus by modulating an L-type calcium conductance. J. Neurosci. 23:816-825.
[58] Albin RL, Young AB, Penney JB (1989) The functional anatomy of basal ganglia disorders. Trends Neurosci. 12:366-375.
[59] Bevan MD, Atherton JF, Baufreton J. (2006) Cellular principles underlying normal and pathological activity in the subthalamic nucleus. Curr. Opin. Neurobiol. 16:621-628.
[60] Hollerman JR, Grace AA (1992) Subthalamic nucleus cell firing in the 6-OHDA-treated rat: basal activity and response to haloperidol. Brain Res. 590:291-299.
[61] Hassani OK, Mouroux M, Féger J. (1996) Increased subthalamic neuronal activity after nigral dopaminergic lesion independent of disinhibition via the globus pallidus. Neuroscience. 72:105-115.
[62] Benazzouz A, Boraud T, Féger J, Burbaud P, Bioulac B, Gross C (1996) Alleviation of experimental hemiparkinsonism by high-frequency stimulation of the subthalamic nucleus in primates: a comparison with L-Dopa treatment. Mov. Disord. 11:627-632.
[63] Rodriguez MC, Guridi OJ, Alvarez L, Mewes K, Macias R, Vitek J, DeLong MR, Obeso JA (1998) The subthalamic nucleus and tremor in Parkinson's disease. Mov. Disord. 3:111-118.
[64] Ammari R, Bioulac B, Garcia L, Hammond C (2011) The Subthalamic Nucleus becomes a Generator of Bursts in the Dopamine-Depleted State. Its High Frequency Stimulation Dramatically Weakens Transmission to the Globus Pallidus. Front. Syst. Neurosci. 5:43.
[65] Garcia L, D'Alessandro G, Bioulac B, Hammond C (2005) High-frequency stimulation in Parkinson's disease: more or less? Trends Neurosci. 28:209-216.

[66] Tai CH, Yang YC, Pan MK, Huang CS, Kuo CC (2011) Modulation of subthalamic T-type Ca(2+) channels remedies locomotor deficits in a rat model of Parkinson disease. J. Clin. Invest. 121:3289-3305.

[67] Zhong G, Díaz-Ríos M, Harris-Warrick RM (2006) Intrinsic and functional differences among commissural interneurons during fictive locomotion and serotonergic modulation in the neonatal mouse. J. Neurosci. 6:6509-6517

[68] Zhong G, Masino MA, Harris-Warrick RM (2007) Persistent sodium currents participate in fictive locomotion generation in neonatal mouse spinal cord. J. Neurosci. 27:4507-18.

[69] Tazerart S, Vinay L, Brocard F (2008) The persistent sodium current generates pacemaker activities in the central pattern generator for locomotion and regulates the locomotor rhythm. J. Neurosci. 28:8577-8589.

[70] Song Y, Li HM, Xie RG, Yue ZF, Song XJ, Hu SJ, Xing JL (2012) Evoked bursting in injured Aβ dorsal root ganglion neurons: a mechanism underlying tactile allodynia. Pain. 153:657-665.

[71] Yao H, Donnelly DF, Ma C, LaMotte RH (2003) Upregulation of the hyperpolarization-activated cation current after chronic compression of the dorsal root ganglion. J. Neurosci. 23:2069-2074.

[72] Jiang YQ, Sun Q, Tu HY, Wan Y (2008) Characteristics of HCN channels and their participation in neuropathic pain. Neurochem. Res. 33:1979-1989.

[73] Yang RH, Xing JL, Duan JH, Hu SJ (2005) Effects of gabapentin on spontaneous discharges and subthreshold membrane potential oscillation of type A neurons in injured DRG. Pain. 116:187-193.

[74] Yang RH, Wang WT, Chen JY, Xie RG, Hu SJ (2009) Gabapentin selectively reduces persistent sodium current in injured type-A dorsal root ganglion neurons. Pain. 143:48-55.

[75] Xie RG, Zheng DW, Xing JL, Zhang XJ, Song Y, Xie YB, Kuang F, Dong H, You SW, Xu H, Hu SJ (2011) Blockade of persistent sodium currents contributes to the riluzole-induced inhibition of spontaneous activity and oscillations in injured DRG neurons. PLoS One. 6:e18681.

[76] Smith JC, Ellenberger HH, Ballanyi K, Richter DW, Feldman JL (1991) Pre-Bötzinger complex: a brainstem region that generate respiratory rhythm in mammals. Science. 254:726-729.

[77] Onimaru H, Homma I (2003) A novel functional neuron group for respiratory rhythm generation in the ventral medulla. J. Neurosci. 23:1478-1486.

[78] Janczewski WA, Feldman JL (2006) Distinct rhythm generators for inspiration and expiration in the juvenile rat. J. Physiol. 570:407-420.

[79] Peña F (2009) Neuronal network properties underlying the generation of gasping. Clin. Exp. Pharmacol. Physiol. 36:1218-1228.

[80] Thoby-Brisson M, Ramirez JM (2001) Identification of two types of inspiratory pacemaker neurons in the isolated respiratory neural network of mice. J. Neurophysiol. 86:104-112.

[81] Del Negro CA, Morgado-Valle C, Feldman JL (2002) Respiratory rhythm: an emergent network property? Neuron. 34(5):821-830.

[82] Del Negro CA, Morgado-Valle C, Hayes JA, Mackay DD, Pace RW, Crowder EA, Feldman JL (2005) Sodium and calcium current-mediated pacemaker neurons and respiratory rhythm generation. J. Neurosci. 25(2):446-453.

[83] Viemari JC, Ramirez JM (2006) Norepinephrine differentially modulates different types of respiratory pacemaker and nonpacemaker neurons. J. Neurophysiol. 95:2070-82.

[84] Tryba AK, Peña F, Ramirez JM (2006) Gasping activity in vitro: a rhythm dependent on 5-HT2A receptors. J. Neurosci. 26:2623-2634.

[85] Mellen NM, Mishra D (2010) Functional anatomical evidence for respiratory rhythmogenic function of endogenous bursters in rat medulla. J. Neurosci. 30:8383-8392.

[86] Ben-Mabrouk F, Tryba AK (2010) Substance P modulation of TRPC3/7 channels improves respiratory rhythm regularity and ICAN-dependent pacemaker activity. Eur. J. Neurosci. 31:1219-1232.

[87] Peña F, Aguileta MA (2007) Effects of riluzole and flufenamic acid on eupnea and gasping of neonatal mice in vivo. Neurosci. Lett. 415:288-293.

[88] Poets CF, Meny RG, Chobanian MR, Bonofiglo RE (1999) Gasping and other cardiorespiratory patterns during sudden infant deaths. Pediatr. Res. 45:350-354.

[89] Sridhar R, Thach BT, Kelly DH, Henslee JA (2003) Characterization of successful and failed autoresuscitation in human infants, including those dying of SIDS. Pediatr. Pulmonol. 36:113-122.

Chapter 7

# Motor Unit Action Potential Duration: Measurement and Significance

Ignacio Rodríguez-Carreño, Luis Gila-Useros and Armando Malanda-Trigueros

Additional information is available at the end of the chapter

http://dx.doi.org/10.5772/50265

## 1. Introduction

The quantification of the bioelectric phenomena originating in nervous and muscular tissues is an essential task in diagnosis within the field of Electromedicine. Clinical electromyography is the part of Clinical Neurophysiology focused on the neuromuscular system, and includes the study of the electrical activity of peripheral nerves (electroneurography), striated muscles (electromyography, in its strict sense) and a number of reflex circuits (reflexology), among others [1].

The background to all these scientific areas is based on the parameterization of the bioelectrical functions of the neuromuscular structures. The definition and formulation of such parameters represents the theoretical and practical basis which enables the analysis of the function of muscles and nerves in normal and pathological conditions. The quantification of bioelectrical parameters makes possible to delimit their normal ranges. The presence of parameter values beyond normal ranges, as measured by neurophysiologic techniques, is used in the diagnosis of diseases of nerves and muscles, which is the main goal of clinical electromyography [2].

A basic concept in electromyography is the so called motor unit (MU), which represents the anatomical and functional element of the neuromuscular system. The MU is formed by the alpha spinal motorneuron and its innervated set of muscular cells. The electrical changes generated by activity of the MU can be acquired and amplified by electrodes located in muscle mass and these changes can be recorded and edited using electromyographic (EMG) devices. The representation of the changes generated by a MU is the so called motor unit action potential (MUAP). A MUAP waveform can be characterized by a number of parameters related to certain aspects of the structure and physiology of the MU (Figure 1). Therefore, the quantitative measurement of such parameters is a basic issue in electromyography, and the duration of the MUAP is a key measure as it defines the boundaries of the MUAP waveform and the rest of the MUAP parameters are measured within the time span defined by the MUAP duration [3].

The main parameters defined to characterize the MUAP waveform are reviewed in this chapter, which also covers the particular issues related to the significance and measurement of the MUAP duration.

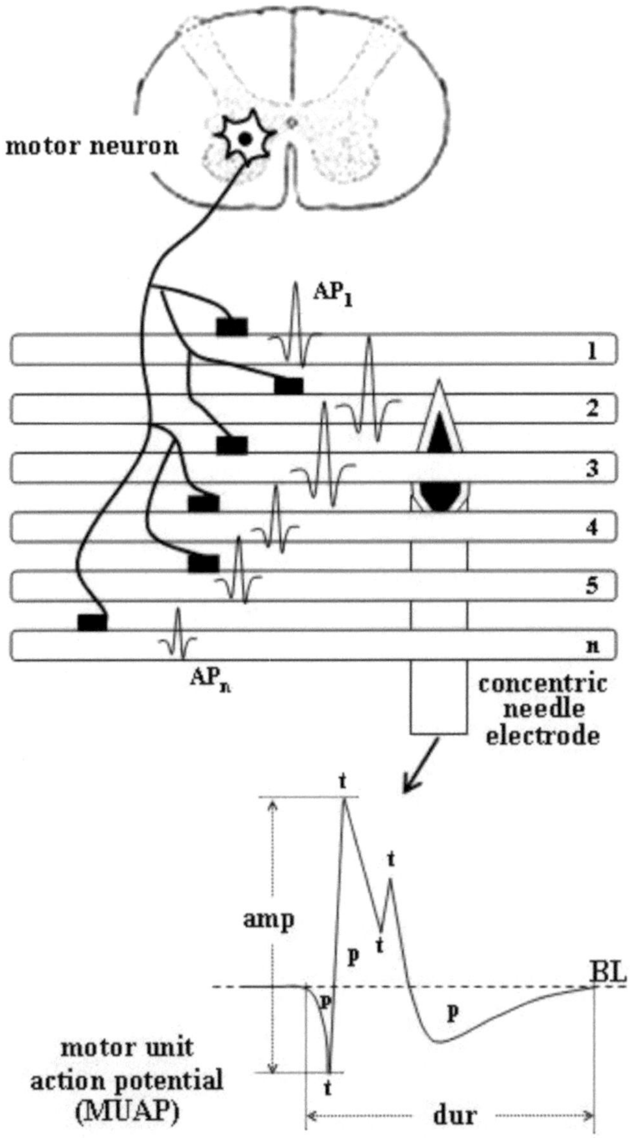


**Figure 1.** Schematic representation of a motor unit with n muscle fibers. The algebraic summation of the action potentials (AP) of all the single fibers present in the recording uptake area of the electrode (AP1+AP2+...+APn) generates the motor unit action potential (MUAP). The main parameters of the MUAP waveform are indicated: amp = amplitude; dur = duration; p = phase; t = turn. BL = baseline.

## 2. Quantitative characterization of MUAP

### 2.1. Anatomical and physiological description of MU and MUAP

Striated or skeletal muscles are the effectors of voluntary movements. Striated muscle cells or muscle fibers (MF) have an elongated form, and their contraction is brought about by the sliding of contractile protein filaments contained in their cytoplasm (sarcoplasm). As in any living cell, across the membrane of MFs there exists a difference of electric potential of approximately 90 mV (the inside of the cell being negative with respect to the outside) because there is a difference in the amount of electrical charge in intra- and extra-cellular fluids. A basic property of MFs and neurons is the ability to change the membrane potential and transiently convert their inside into a positive potential in specific conditions. This inversion of potential or depolarization is called an action potential (AP), and it arises by a brief opening of membrane sodium channels, with the consequent rise in the membrane permeability to this ion. The changes of ionic fluxes related to the AP are transmitted towards neighbouring points of the membrane, being conducted along the MF at a velocity of 3-5 m/s. After the depolarization begins, the repolarization phase proceeds, in which there is further passive and active (by the action of the Na-K pump) transmembrane flux of ions, which restores the basal conditions of the membrane at rest. [4].

The nervous system controls the degree of contraction of the MFs by means of the frequency of the nervous impulses of the alpha motor neurons, whose central cellular components are located in the anterior horns of the spinal cord. These nervous impulses are APs of the motor neurons; they travel along the axons and are transmitted to MFs at neuromuscular junctions. As previously described, the system formed by an alpha motor neuron and its set of innervated MFs forms a MU, which represents the anatomical and functional unit of skeletal muscle. The number of MFs innervated by the MU varies according to the muscle. The number is small in the eye muscles, that need very precise adjustments; the large muscles of the lower extremities have several hundred MFs [5]. During a slight voluntary contraction, only a few MUs are activated, and they discharge APs at low frequencies (around 5 per second). To increase the strength of contraction, the nervous system drives a progressive increase in the discharge frequency and a progressive activation or recruitment of other MUs in the muscle concerned.

The recording and analysis of the electrical activity of MFs and MUs (myoelectrical activity) is the subject of electromyography. Conventional EMG studies are performed with needle electrodes that capture the activity of MFs within a hemisphere of 2.5 mm radius from the tip of the needle electrode. To study the MUAPs of a certain muscle, a needle electrode is inserted into the muscle mass, which the subject is asked to maintain under slight contraction. In this way, a low number of MUs are activated and the successive discharges of the corresponding MUAPs can be collected. If the degree of contraction is excessive, too many MUs are discharging and the recorded waveforms of their MUAPs are distorted by their superposition.

In Europe, the needle electrodes currently used are concentric, which have a core of platinum or stainless steel embedded in insulating material located inside a stainless steel cannula. The core is the active electrode, and the cannula is the reference electrode. A MUAP is a recording of the changes produced by the discharge of the MFs of a MU (Figure 1). In general, normal MUAPs show mean peak-to-peak amplitudes of around 0.5 mV and a duration from 8 to 14 ms, depending on the size of the MUs. The size and shape of MUAPs is determined by certain structural and functional aspects of MUs. Pathologic processes of the peripheral nervous system (neurogenic processes) and of muscles (myopathic pathologies) can alter these aspects, leading to abnormal deviations in MUAP parameters; i.e., the EMG signal captures pathologic remodelling of the MUs caused by neuromuscular diseases. Once other neurophysiologic data and the clinical context of the patient have been taken into account, a deviation with respect to the normal pattern for a given muscle constitutes the basis of an EMG diagnosis.

## 2.2. Parameters of the MUAP and their physiological significance

To characterize a MUAP waveform quantitatively, a number of parameters have been defined (Figure 1). These parameters are related to certain anatomical and physiological aspects of MFs and MUs. There are three groups of MUAP parameters to characterize the size, shape and stability, respectively, of the MUAP. These parameters, which provide information about certain spatial and temporal characteristics of MF and MU activity, are described below:

1. Size parameters are related to the size (diameter), number and density of generators of a MUAP (i.e. the MFs of the MU). These parameters include duration, amplitude, area and indices such as the size index and thickness index. Since duration will be treated extensively later in this chapter, it will not be described in this section, where a brief description of the other parameters is given.

The amplitude is the voltage difference from minimum to maximum peaks. Computer simulations of MUAPs show that the amplitude is determined by the few MFs (less than eight) located within a semicircular uptake area of 0.5 mm radius from the electrode [6]. Consequently, amplitude can vary considerably within the MU territory (the space within which the MFs of a MU are randomly scattered).

Area can be calculated automatically by integrating the rectified MUAP within the duration. It depends on the MFs present within 1.5 mm from the core of the concentric electrode [7]. Relatively small movements of the recording electrode affect the amplitude and area parameters considerably because the amplitude of the APs of the MFs decays quickly with distance to the electrode [8].

In the quest for more stable estimators of the magnitude of MU generators, new parameters have been defined, the most relevant being the thickness and size indices. The thickness index is computed as the area-to-amplitude ratio, and is a sensitive detector of myopathic abnormalities [9], but not of neurogenic ones. To improve detection of neurogenic MUAPs, multivariate analysis was used to find the optimal separation from normal MUAPs; in this way, the size index was formulated as [2 x $\log_{10}$ (amplitude) + (area/amplitude)]. However, this index is not significantly better than other parameters for the detection of abnormality in myopathic conditions [10].

2. MUAP waveform shape parameters transcribe the temporal synchrony / dispersion of the activation times of the MFs and their conduction velocities. These parameters include the number of phases, the number of turns, and indices such as the coefficient of irregularity.

A phase is the part of a MUAP that falls between two baseline (BL) crossings. A turn is a peak (i.e. a point of directional change) in a MUAP waveform. The number of phases is counted within the MUAP duration. Various amplitude and duration criteria are used in computerized measurements to exclude from the count brief BL crossings or small peaks, which may be due to noise [11]. Normal MUAPs have simple shapes between two and four phases. Polyphasic MUAPs have more than four phases, and those with more than five turns are called polyturn or complex MUAPs. These terms all reflect the same feature: increased temporal dispersion of MFs potentials, but polyphasia indicates more pronounced changes.

To enhance the sensitivity and precision of measurement of MF synchronicity, other estimators have been proposed, such as the coefficient of irregularity [12]. This is defined as the total amplitude change (over the MUAP length) divided by the peak-to-peak amplitude. The minimum value that MUAP irregularity can have is 2. As the complexity of a waveform increases, the value of this index increases too. Significant differences have been found between pathologies (neurogenic as well as myopathic) of both slow and quick progression [13]; but in general, and in spite of its theoretical background, the coefficient of irregularity has not shown better performance than conventional parameters.

3. Stability parameters or jiggle parameters have been defined to quantify the degree of variability in MUAP shape at consecutive discharges [14]. These parameters are the consecutive amplitude differences (CAD) and cross-correlational coefficients of consecutive discharges (CCC). The efficiency of CAD and CCC has been proved mainly in simulated signals. There are very few studies with real EMG recordings [15], but the presence of noise has been found to significantly affect quantification of the jiggle using these parameters, and consequently the estimation of jiggle still requires subjective verification by visual assessment.

## 3. MUAP duration

### 3.1. Definition

MUAP duration is defined as the time from the start of activation of MU fibers until the end of their repolarization phase, i.e., the time in which the bioelectric changes produced by a discharge of a MU take place.

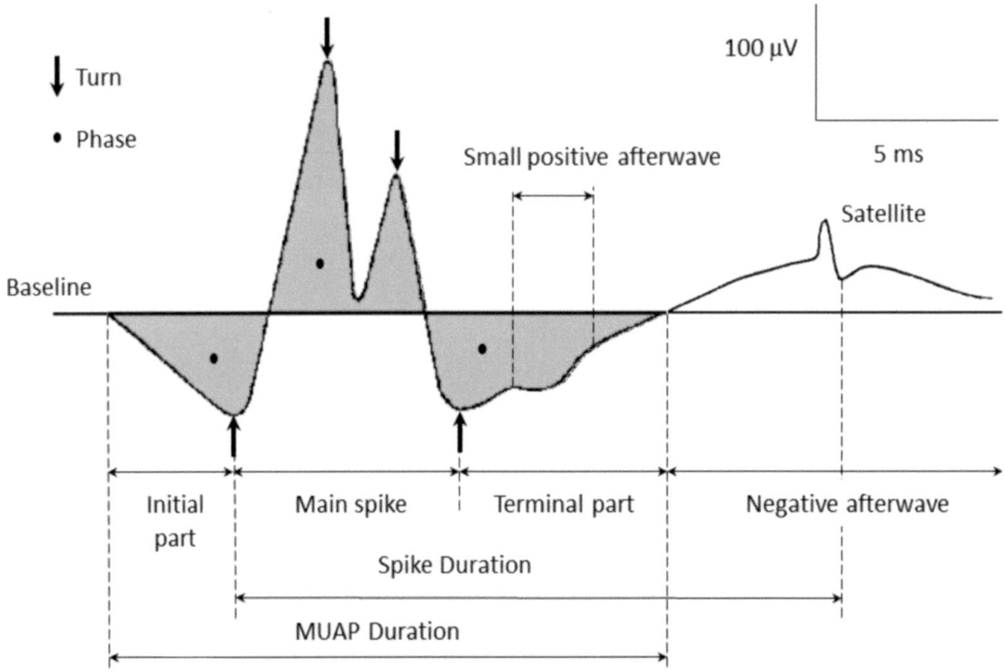


**Figure 2.** Parts of the MUAP. MUAP parameters: duration, spike duration, turns, phases.

## 3.2. Parts of the MUAP

Over the duration of a MUAP, several parts of the MUAP waveform can be delimited (Figure 2), each one having specific structural and functional significance [16]:

1. The initial part: from the start of MF activation to the first positive turn. Graphically this is a positive deflection whose charactersitics depend on the distance of the motor end-plate region until the situation of the recording electrode in the length of the fiber. If the electrode is close to the end-plate zone, the initial positive part in the MUAP hardly exists, and the MUAP waveform begins with an initial upward defection (Figure 3). As the distance between the end-plate region and the tip of the electrode increases, the initial part becomes more and more evident and its duration increases as well, being maximal when the electrode is located near the extreme of the MFs near the tendon. [3, 16-18].
2. The spike part: between the first and the last positive turns. The spike part mainly depends on the temporal dispersion of the MF potentials as they pass in the vicinity of the recording electrode. It is thought likely that only less than 15 fibers contribute to the spike part in normal MUs [19]. The spike usually has one negative peak, called the main spike, but may have several positive peaks. Note that a MUAP may contain spike components other than the main spike. Such parts are called satellites. Spike duration is measured between the first and the last positive peak of the MUAP (Figure 2). If the MUAP is recorded in the end-plate region, the start of the MUAP and of the spike part coincide, because there is no initial part. The spike duration is usually shorter than the

total duration, but this does not need necessarily be so if a satellite is present. Satellites, which usually follow the terminal part (but exceptionally precede the initial part), are included in the measurement of spike duration and thus, spike duration may exceed the total duration of the MUAP [20].

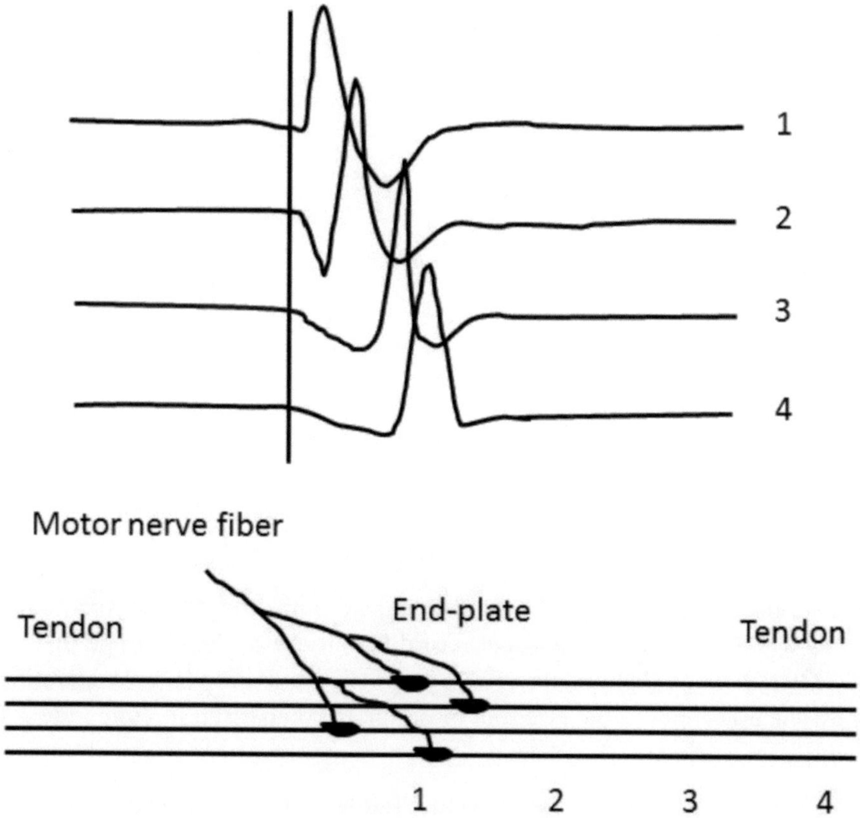


**Figure 3.** Example of recording a MUAP at different distances from the end-plate zone (position 1). As the distance from the end plate increases (1 to 4), the initial positive part of the MUAP becomes longer. Below, a schematic presentation of the recording positions with respect to the end-plate zone.

3. The terminal part: from the last positive turn until the endpoint, where the signal reaches the BL. The terminal part is longer than the previous parts because the approach to the BL is gradual. The terminal part is generated by the volley of APs leaving the electrode and it includes the main part of the repolarization phase.
4. Small positive afterwave: these are not usually seen in recordings with concentric electrodes, but can be observed within the terminal part of MUAPs in recordings performed with monopolar electrodes (which are more commonly used in the United States than Europe). The small positive afterwave reflects the arrival of MF depolarization at the muscle-tendon union with the tendon [21]. When a small positive wave is present, usually superimposed on the terminal part, it is included in the MUAP duration.

5. Negative afterwave: this is an artifactual wave that arises due to the effect of the high-pass filter of the amplifier (Figure 4), mainly when the MUAP has a dominating positive phase, which is counterbalanced by a negative afterwave [22, 23]. A negative afterwave usually has low amplitude (less than 10 microvolts), but, in any case, it is an artifact and should be excluded from duration measurements.

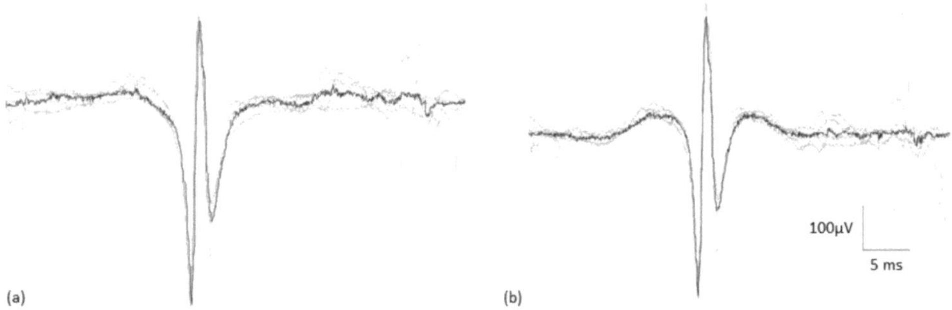


**Figure 4.** Effects of the high pass filter in the MUAP waveform. The cut-off frequencies of the filters 8 applied in (a) and (b) are 10 and 50 Hz, respectively.

### 3.3. Physiopathological significance of MUAP duration

Computer simulations of the MUAP indicate that the duration reflects the current generated by the MFs within 2.5 mm of the active recording surface of the electrode [6]. The total current is determined by the number of MFs and their cross-sectional area. Duration is not affected by slight changes in the electrode position, in comparison to amplitude and area, both of which are sensitive to this change.

The total MUAP duration comprises the slow initial and terminal phases of the MUAP signal. These parts represent the time when the APs of the MFs are at some distance from the electrode and the APs are still relatively equidistant from the recording surface and contribute to a similar extent. Therefore, the duration of the normal MUAP is not so much dependent on the temporal dispersion of the individual MF APs but more on the number of MFs within the recording area [3]. Although the degree of temporal dispersion of the APs of MFs is specifically expressed by the spike duration and shape parameters, temporal dispersion also influences the magnitude of the total MUAP duration, as can be seen in pathologic MUAPs. When there is large variability in MF diameters, an enlarged end-plate region or a mixture of slow- and fast-conducting terminal axons, the temporal dispersion of MF potentials is pronounced, resulting in MUAPs with long durations and more or less complex waveforms (sometimes extremely complex).

The physiopathological correlations underlying the magnitude of total MUAP duration, makes the duration measurement clinically useful (Table 1). The duration is a parameter currently used in clinical electromyography and its normative values have been established over samples of normal subjects for each muscle and age range. [24, 25]. Reference values from healthy subjects show little correlation to gender, height and weight. Within the age range of 15 to 65 years the effect of age is negligible [26], but an increase of duration has been reported for subjects of older ages [27].

| MUAP abnormality | Anatomical phenomena related |
|---|---|
| *Decreased amplitude* | Muscle fibers' atrophia<br>Increasement of connective tissue<br>Excessive jitter and blocking |
| *Increased amplitude* | Muscle fibers grouping (reinervation, regeneration)<br>Muscle fibers hypertrophia |
| *Decreased duration* | Muscle fibers' atrophia<br>Loss of muscle fibers<br>Serious MUAPs blocking in endplate |
| *Increased duration* | Increase in the number of muscle fibers (collateral growing) |
| *Increased spike duration* | Variation in the diameter of the muscle fibers<br>Increase in the width of the endplate |
| *Increase in the number of turns and phases* | Slow conduction in terminal axons<br>Increase in the width of the endplate<br>Increase in the variability of the diameter of muscle fibers |
| *Increase in the firing rate* | Loss of MUs<br>Decrease in the force generated by individual MUs |
| *Increase in the jiggle* | Abnormal neuromuscular transmission |

**Table 1.** Relation between MUAP alterations and abnormality reflected.

For the EMG examination of a muscle, a sample of 20 MUAPs must be extracted [18]. The mean values of the different MUAP parameters are matched up with their respective reference values. Deviations from normality may be defined as a value of mean duration plus/minus 2 standard deviations above or below that for samples from the normal population for the same muscle and age group as the subject under study [28].

Abnormally high duration values result from an abnormal increase in the number of MFs in the MUs in neurogenic processes due to collateral reinnervation and focal grouping. The neurogenic MUAPs can have simple or complex shapes and can be stable or instable (normal or increased jiggle) depending on the nature of the pathology and its temporal course (acute, subacute or chronic). With regard to abnormally low duration values, a low duration reflects loss of MFs in myopathic processes, myophatic atrophy of MFs or neurogenic lesions at early stages of reinnervation (nascent MUAPs), or severe blocking of neuromuscular transmission (such as in botulism or myasthenia gravis).

MUAP duration is a basic parameter of the MUAP due to its physiopathologic significance and also due to the fact that the duration markers (the established start and end points) define the boundaries of the MUAP waveform and thereby separate those parts of the recorded signal which will be analyzed from other parts, such as BL or background activity. All MUAP parameters and features are measured within the MUAP duration or, in the event of the presence of satellites, with respect to it; consequently, duration is the first parameter that must be determined.

## 4. Measurement of MUAP duration

### 4.1. A challenge for quantitative electromyography

Technical improvements implemented on recent EMG machines have made many aspects of EMG examinations easier. Examples of such improvements are facilities for extraction of MUAP signals; edition, storage, automatic measurement of parameters; calculation of mean values; and the process of matching normative ranges. However, in clinical electromyography, diagnostic judgment, i.e., the final diagnostic conclusions built upon the collected data, is still mainly dependent on the knowledge and experience of the electromyographist who performs the study. Quantitative methods try to overcome subjective considerations by means of precise measurements of physiopathologically significant features. The performance of such methodologies is in general satisfactory when the conditions of the study are favorable: a collaborating patient, a fully developed pathology, and low levels of noise. But, working circumstances are seldom so perfect, and there are still important limitations mainly due to two disrupting factors that currently can only be partially controlled: variability and noise. In this respect, the measurement of MUAP duration can serve as a paradigmatic example of a fundamental challenge facing clinical neurophysiology: how to extract objective and consistent parameter estimates. The nature of the challenge is shown in the following considerations.

### 4.2. Clinical and physiologic duration

The definition of MUAP duration is, as stated above, simply the time between the beginning and the end of the bio-electrical activity of the MUs detected by the recording electrode. Often, the "duration onset" can be easily determined because the takeoff of the MUAP waveform, which is associated with the depolarization of MFs at the end-plates, is so abrupt that the waveform appears clearly deflected from the BL. This occurs especially if the recording has been made close to the end-plate zone and if the MUAP does not have an initial negative part. However, the "duration end", which is not associated with any clearly identified physiological event, is more difficult to determine because the terminal part of the waveform approaches the BL gradually. With real recordings and in simulation studies, it has been demonstrated that the extinction of APs continues for over 20 ms after the main spike of the MUAP [29-31]. In real recordings, a very stable BL and a large number of averaged discharges are needed in order to observe such a slow return to the BL in the terminal part of the MUAP. Routine recordings, however, almost invariably have slow BL fluctuations and other noisy interference that obscure the full extension of the terminal part. Thus, two meanings of "duration" should be considered: the "physiologic" (as defined above) and the "clinical" [29, 30]. The above considerations are indicative of the operational difficulties encountered with the simple physiologic definition of MUAP duration. The concept of clinical duration is that applied generally in diagnostic applications and will be used in the rest of this text. As with physiologic duration, there are difficulties in the measurement of MUAP clinical duration. These difficulties are discussed below.

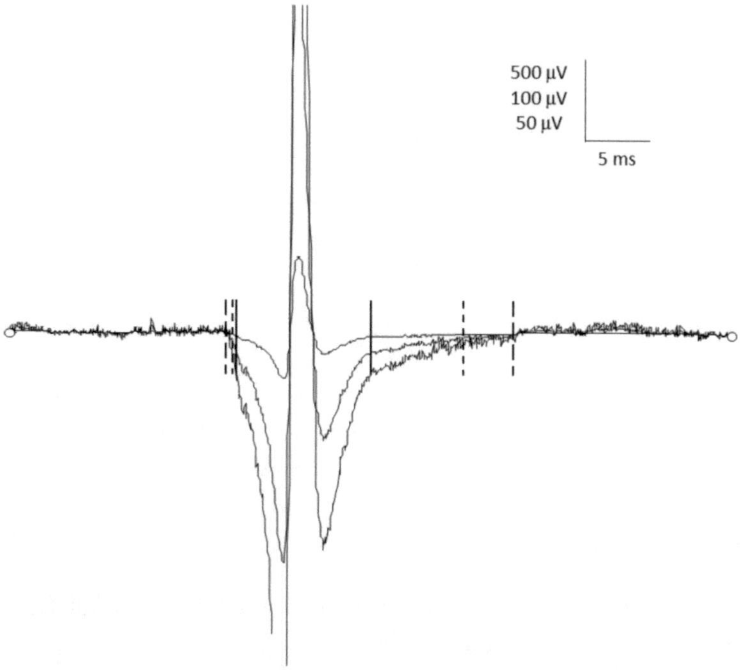


**Figure 5.** The same MUAP displayed at different gains. As the MUAP is amplified, its duration is measured longer due to the visual effect. Continuous, short dashed, and dashed lines represent the duration markers at 500, 100 and 50 μV/cm, respectively.

## 4.3. Manual measurement of clinical MUAP duration

Clinical MUAP duration is defined as the time between the start and end points of the MUAP, when observed at a sensitivity of 100 μV/cm and a sweep screen of 10 ms/cm [3, 16, 29]. At higher gains, duration measurements tend to be longer because more of the slight initial or terminal slopes are visible before they merge with the random noise of background activity [23], see Figure 5. The gain of 100 μ V/cm was arbitrarily chosen to standardize the visual resolution at which duration markers should be manually placed. In this way, duration can be conceived of as a morphological feature, operationally defined in accordance with a specified magnitude of display resolution at which the recorded signal is represented.

When making manual measurements, electromyographists measure MUAP duration by visual inspection at the standardized settings stated above. Manual measurements can be made for an isolated discharge, over the averaged potential resulting from a set of MUAP discharges or by visual inspection of a set of discharges in superimposed and/or raster modes.

### 4.4. Automatic measurement of MUAP duration

A number of algorithmic methods for automatic measurement of duration have been designed and implemented on commercial equipment. Such algorithms aim to reproduce the manual procedure, and those used in computer-aided methods include BL calculation and use quantitative amplitude or slope criterion or a combination of both to look for the limit points between the MUAP waveform and the BL [3, 16]. Quantitative definitions applied to the analysis of morphologic features of the MUAP are similar to the automatic counting of turns and phases [32, 33]. Usually these algorithms are applied to the averaged MUAP waveform obtained from the discharges that have been recorded and extracted with automatic assistance [34, 35].

One might expect these algorithms to be more reliable than manual measurement, but in fact they suffer from several limitations when dealing with real signals. High variability has been observed in automatic as well as manual measurements. In addition, automatic measurements are often inaccurate, always require visual supervision, and frequently require manual correction of duration marker positions.

## 5. Variability of manual measurements

Duration has long been recognized as the most difficult MUAP parameter to define and measure in an unequivocal way, and exact positioning of the endpoint is recognized to be somewhat arbitrary [16]. It is therefore likely that the inter- and intra-examiner variability of manual duration measurements is greater than that for the other MUAP parameters. An important consequence of this variability is that the normal limits of MUAP duration for a given muscle and age range have broad margins, which drastically reduce the diagnostic sensitivity of the parameter [36]. Thus, whilst large deviations from normality are easily identified, the intepretation of the significance of smaller deviations depends considerably on the examiner.

Several studies have investigated the variability of repeated manual duration measurements. In one study, a set of 25 nearly-normal MUAPs recorded from the brachial biceps muscle were manually analyzed three times on different days by the same single electromyographist. In the three repeated manual measurements, the mean durations ranged from 14.9 to 15.7 ms, and the largest difference between durations of MUAPs from the same MU was 8 ms [16]. Similar observations of such low degrees of reliability of manual duration readings have been reported by other authors [37-39].

In another study, for a systematic quantitative estimation of the intra- and inter-examiner variability in MUAP duration measurements, the Gage Reproducibility and Repeatability (Gage R&R) method [40, 41] was applied [42]. This method is based on the analysis of the variance of repeated measurements of a given feature, and it is currently applied in industrial quality control studies. It was designed to assess both the variability in product magnitudes caused by the production process itself (part-to-part variability) and the variability attributable to the measurement system (the gage). The latter component of variability includes that attributable to the measurement device (the repeatability or intraoperator variability), assessed by repeated measurements by the same operator, and that attributable to the operator (reproducibility or interoperator variability), assessed by comparison of the measurements made by different operators. In the context of MUAP duration measurement, the part-to-part variability is related to the intrinsic variability of MUAP duration present in each sample of MUAPs extracted from a given muscle. This intrinsic variability of MUAP duration (i.e. variability of the object being measured as opposed to the process of measurement) is due to differences in size and structure of a muscle's MUs and to differences in electrode positioning within the muscle.

The Gage R&R method was applied to six independent duration measurements performed by two electromyographists (three measurements separated in time by each electromyographist) on a set of 240 MUAPs from two muscles without pathology: the tibialis anterior and the first dorsal interosseous. The MUAPs accepted for analysis had well-defined waveforms and were free of superposition, gross BL fluctuations and distortions of other sources. In order to make manual measurements, an interactive software tool displaying the averaged MUAP and the set of the extracted discharges in raster and superimposed modes was provided. The time base and sensitivity could be changed by the operators, but the sensitivity and sweep speed for placing duration markers was fixed at the standard values of 100 μV/cm and 10 ms/cm, respectively.

In spite of the favourable conditions (the clean and well-defined MUAP waveforms and the good-quality visualization and measurement software), a high degree of variability in duration measurements was observed. Of the six evaluations of start marker position, the biggest difference for a MUAP was 6.6 ms. Broader ranges, up to 11.2 ms, were observed for end marker positions. The biggest ranges were observed in end marker positions for MUAPs with a long and gradually-sloped terminal part to their waveforms (Figure 6a). This particular feature of MUAP waveforms was found to be the major cause of difficulty in the manual procedure, since other confounding factors, such as the presence of noise, BL fluctuations and secondary MUAPs in the recordings, were minimised at the time of selecting samples of MUAPs for the study. Examples of other difficulties encountered in manual placement of duration markers are given in Figure 6.

The reproducibility and repeatability analysis by the Gage R&R method decomposes the total variability of the measurements into that intrinsic to the sampled MUAPs (the part-to-part variability, i.e., the variability in the measured parameter *per se*) and the variability attributable to the electromyographists. The latter component accounted for over 30% of total variability and was mainly due to variability in repeated measurements by the same examiner (intraoperator variability). In industrial contexts, where the Gage R&R method is frequently used, degrees of operator variability greater than 10% are considered as poor, and greater than 30% as unacceptable [43].

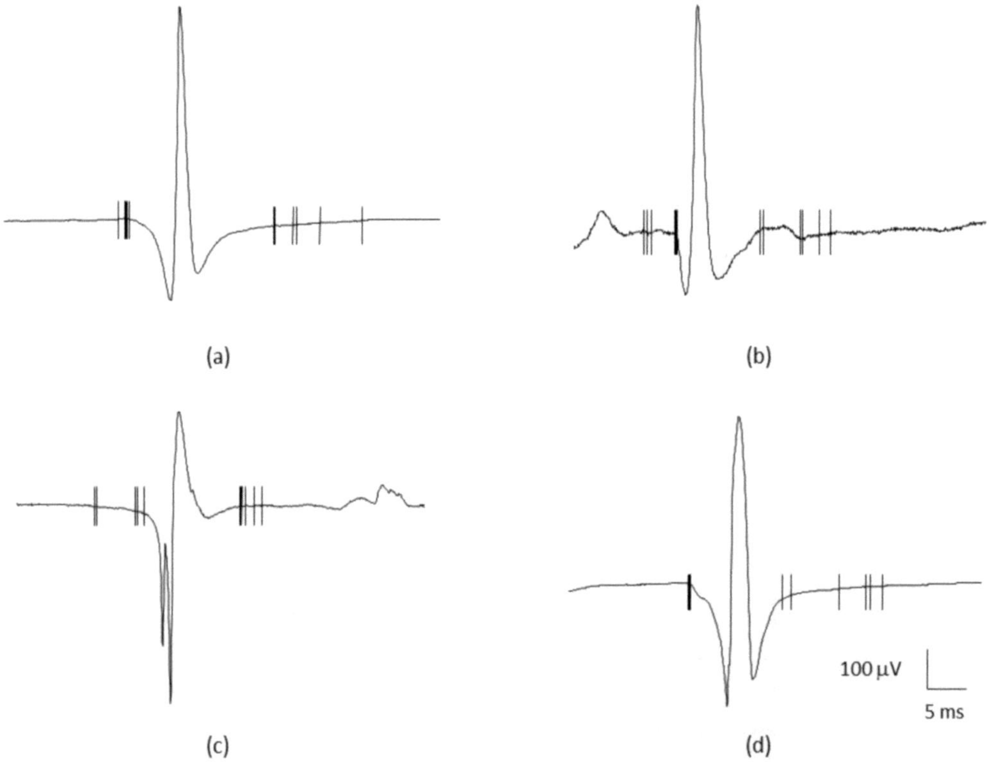


**Figure 6.** Variability in the manual placement of the duration markers. For different electromyographists, there are usually small differences in the manual positions of the start markers (a, d). Great dispersion in the position of the start or end marker can be seen occasionally in the initial part of the MUAP when it has a low slope (a, c). Superimposed discharges of other MUAPs over the initial or terminal portions of the MUAP waveform (b) and the presence of two different slopes separated by an inflexion point at the final portion of the MUAP (d) can be other sources of greta variability in the position of end marker.

## 6. Proposal of a "gold standard" for MUAP duration measurement

As can be concluded from the above discussion, a manual procedure does not guarantee consistent and reliable measurements of MUAP duration. Therefore, if duration markers are automatically placed by a modern EMG device and an error is detected by visual inspection, manual correction does not ensure an accurate estimate of MUAP duration.

In order to assess the effectiveness of a given automatic method of MUAP duration measurement, it is necessary to have available a "gold standard" of duration marker positions (GSP), that is, the marker positions which the automatic method should be finding automatically. Since, as a result of the conceptual and operational limitations exposed above, no single manual measurement can be accepted as the true and exact one, a probabilistic approach to the definition of the GSP has been proposed [42]. For the start or end point of a given MUAP, the GSP was calculated from a set of six marker positions obtained from the repeated marker placements made by two examiners. Specifically, the GSP was calculated as the mean of the three marker positions that were closest together.

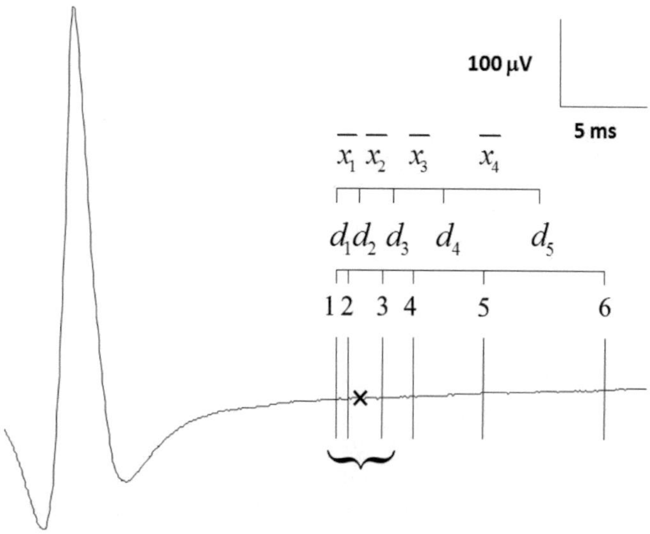


**Figure 7.** Determination of the gold standard of the GSP in an example of six manual marker positions of the end point.

As illustrated in the example in Figure 7, the six markers were ordered by their respective time values from lesser to greater (1 to 6). The five differences between the six position values were obtained ($d_1$ to $d_5$) and the means between two consecutive differences were calculated ( $\bar{x}_1$ to $\bar{x}_4$ ). The smallest of the four mean values was selected ( $\bar{x}_1$ in this example) and the GSP (marked with a cross in the figure) was obtained as the mean of the three manual markers with lowest mean difference (markers 1, 2 and 3 in this example) [42]. By means of this approximation, although a position cannot be assumed to be "true" or even "the best", it can be regarded as a "most likely" position. Thus, such a position can be adopted as a GSP on the basis that it is better in a probabilistic sense than any single position made by manual placement.

## 7. Description of conventional methods for automatic measurement of MUAP duration

The use of computer-aided measurements can theoretically resolve the problem of intra- and inter-examiner variability. The execution of any algorithm on the same signal will always give the same results, without any variability in repeated measurements. In view of this, several automatic methods were developed to try to reproduce the manual procedure used by electromyographists, using amplitude and/or slope criteria to look for the limit points of the MUAP waveform with respect to the BL. Among the reported methods there are differences in several aspects, as described in detail in [16] and [35]. To illustrate these computer-aided techniques, a brief description of several conventional automatic methods (CAMs) is given below. Descriptions include a consideration of differences in the extraction procedure of the MUAP waveform, the definition of the BL and the criteria applied to find the MUAP start and end points (the duration markers positions). The five methods reviewed are the Turku method 1 (T1), the Turku method 2 (T2), the Uppsala method 2 (U2), the Aalborg method (AM) [16], and the Nandedkar's method (NM) [35].

The methods calculate the MUAP duration within a 40, 50 or 100 ms long analysis window. MUAP waveform extraction procedure differ in the following ways:

- In T1 and T2, MUAPs are manually isolated with a trigger level. To reduce high frequency noise and the effect of the presence of other MUAPs in the analysis window, 100 discharges are averaged.
- In AM, MUAPs are automatically isolated and classified by a template matching method using the main spike of the potential. From the set of discharges of the same MUAP, the three most similar ones are selected to obtain the averaged waveform.
- In U2, MUAPs are manually isolated, and the MUAP waveform is obtained by averaging between 20 and 200 discharges.
- In NM, MUAPs are automatically isolated, identified and classified using a multi-MUAP system. From 50 to 65 discharges are extracted for each MUAP, and the MUAP waveform is obtained using median averaging.

With respect to definition of the BL and the MUAP start and end markers, the different criteria used by the five automatic methods are outlined below:

- In T1 and T2, the BL is the average of samples at both 3 and 4 ms ends of the analysis window. NM calculates the BL as the average of the first 5 ms. U2 and AM calculate the BL as the electrical zero.
- Once the BL has been subtracted, T1 and U2 begin their searches for the start and end of the MUAP from the start and end of the analysis window, respectively. T2 and AM begin their searches from a triggering point in the rising slope of the main spike. NM begins its search from the maximum peak.
- T1, T2, AM and U2 use thresholds related to the amplitude/slope values of individual samples or windows of samples (Figure 8a). NM uses thresholds related to the area under the MUAP and to the amplitude sample values (Figure 8b).

## 8. Accuracy of conventional automatic methods

Automatic measurements are free of the intra- and inter-examiner variability present in manual measurements. On ideal EMG signals with well-defined waveforms and without noise, the algorithms may perform satisfactorily. But on real recordings, the available methods for automatic measurement of MUAP duration demonstrate poor agreement and low stability [32]. Thus, visual inspection is always necessary and manual cursor adjustments are frequently required. This is the everyday experience in clinical practice;

And it has been reported by various authors that manual correction of automatic placements is required for 20-50% of MUAPs [26, 34, 38, 44].

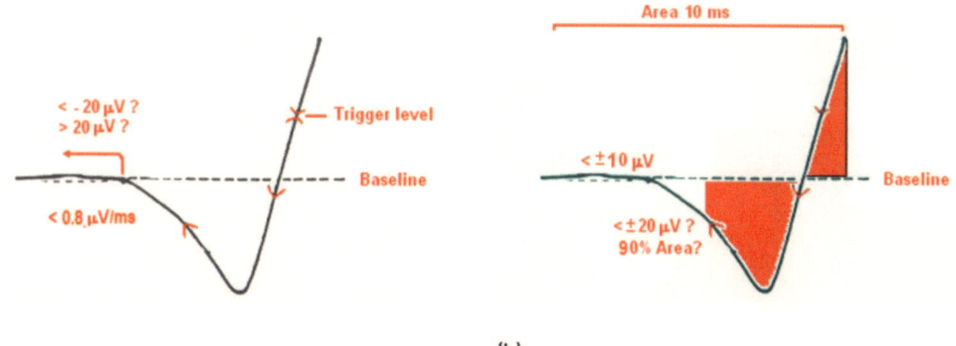


(a) (b)

**Figure 8.** Description T2 and NM. In T2 (a), the MUAP onset is determined from the trigger to a point with slope < 0.8 μV/ms over a 1 ms. If there is a point before with amplitude > 20 μV, a new point fulfilling the slope criterion is looked for. In NM (b), the peak with maximum deviation from the BL is identified. The area of the MUAP from the first sample to the peak is calculated. Then the sample point with 90% of this area to the peak is obtained. If the absolute amplitude at this point is greater than 20 μV, a sample with 10 μV amplitude towards the beginning of the window will be the MUAP onset. Otherwise a point toward the peak with 20 μV amplitude is reached. The MUAP onset then will be the point with amplitude 10 μV toward the first sample.

The accuracy of CAMs has been systematically assessed in normal and pathological MUAPs [42] [45]. Comparing the GSPs (determined by means of the probabilistic method referred above) with the marker positions obtained with CAMs (Figure 9), mean differences of up to 8.5 ms were found, with the T1 CAM. Absolute differences of more than 5 ms between the GSP and an automatic marker position (considered gross errors) were found in many cases: from 15.0% for AM end markers to 49.6% for U2 end markers.

In pathological MUAPs, the worst CAM results were observed with chronic neurogenic MUAPs, which have unusually long duration and are highly polyphasic (Figure 10c and 10d). The results were slightly better with myopathic (Figure 10a) and subacute neurogenic MUAPs (Figure 10b). Analysis of the mean and standard deviation of differences to the GSP (bias and precision, respectively) of the CAMs, showed that some methods, particularly the NM method, provided relatively good results with some pathologic MUAP groups. However, rates of gross errors (differences greater than 5 ms) were seen in around 40% of estimates for several pathologic groups.

In general, end marker placement presents higher levels of error than start marker placement. As in the manual procedure, errors in end marker placement are more pronounced for MUAPs with long-tailed terminal parts. (Figure 10c). Other important sources of error that reduce the performance of CAMs are the presence of several kinds of noise in the recordings, such as the superposition of secondary MUAPs over the analyzed MUAP or BL, and BL fluctuations (Figure 9a. 9b, 9c).

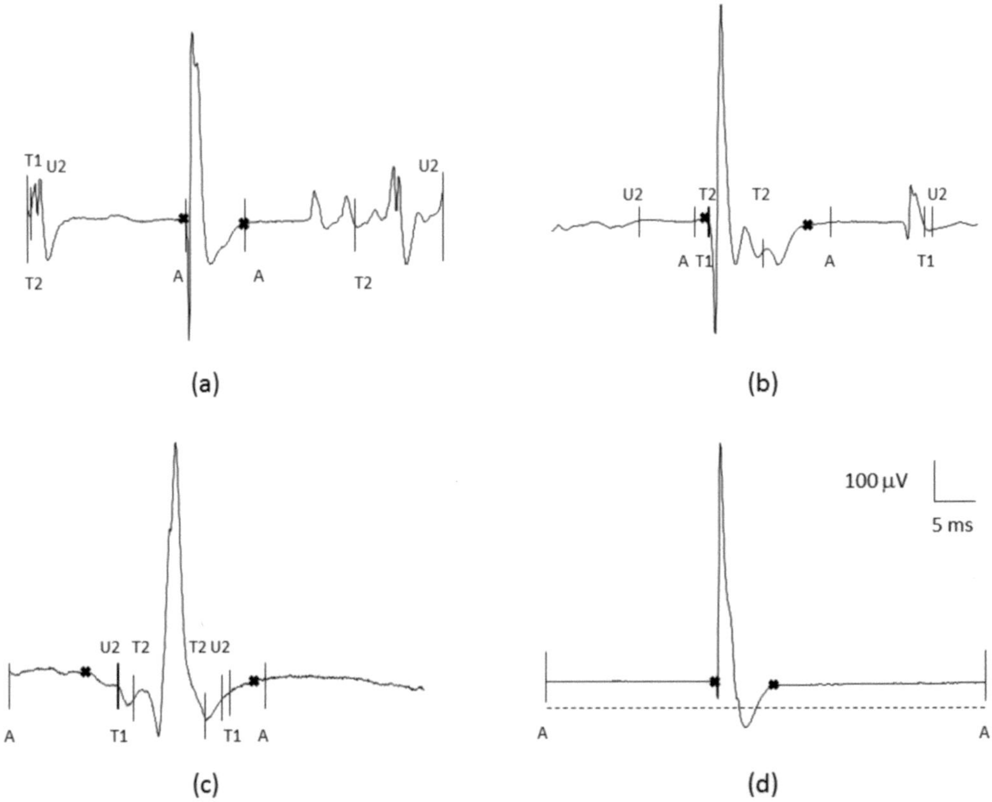


**Figure 9.** CAMs Errors in normal MUAPs. The presence of discharges of secondary MUAPs upon the BL before or after the analysed MUAP waveform induces gross errors in U2 and T1 (a and b). Distortions of the MUAP waveform may cause errors in automatic placements (start markers in c). Poor agreement can be seen among the automatic end marker placements in MUAPs with relatively slow terminal slope (c). Misplacements can also result from an inadequate estimation of the BL, calculated as a constant value, electrical zero in Aalborg method (d).

An attempt to improve the performance of CAMs was carried out by means a signal process to accommodate BL fluctuation [46]. Conceptually, the EMG signal may be considered as an isoelectric BL (zero value) in which the discharges of the active MUs are superimposed. But in real recordings, the BL always shows slow fluctuations due to the activity of distant MUs and movements of the needle electrode. Two problems arise: on the one hand, the high-pass filter does not fully clean all the slow fluctuation and, on the other hand, if the high-pass filter's cut-off frequency is too high, the MUAP waveform can be distorted by creation of a more or less prominent negative afterwave, as previously described. The conventional approaches for dealing with the BL, are either to regard the BL as a straight line [23] of zero value (used by the U2 and AM methods) or to regard the BL as the average of the samples in initial and final segments of the analysis window (used by T1, T2 and NM methods) [16, 35]. An alternative approach for cancelling the BL fluctuation is to reconstruct the course of the BL followed by specific filtering designed not to distort the MUAP waveform [46]. For this purpose, standard methods as adaptive filters have been found unsatisfactory. The sequential application of several techniques of signal processing was necessary, including: 1) wavelet transforms for identifying segments of the EMG signal free of MUAP discharges, 2) averaging of the samples of each of these segments, 3) reconstruction of curves through the averaged points using cubic splines, 4) frequency analysis of this reconstructed BL, and 5) specific filtering based on autoregressive (AR) modeling. In spite of the sophisticated cancellation of BL fluctuation demonstrated by this method, the MUAP duration results of the five CAMs evaluated were not significantly improved when they were provided with signals that had been submitted to it [47]. To optimize automatic duration measurement, strategies other than, or in addition to, BL treatment are required.

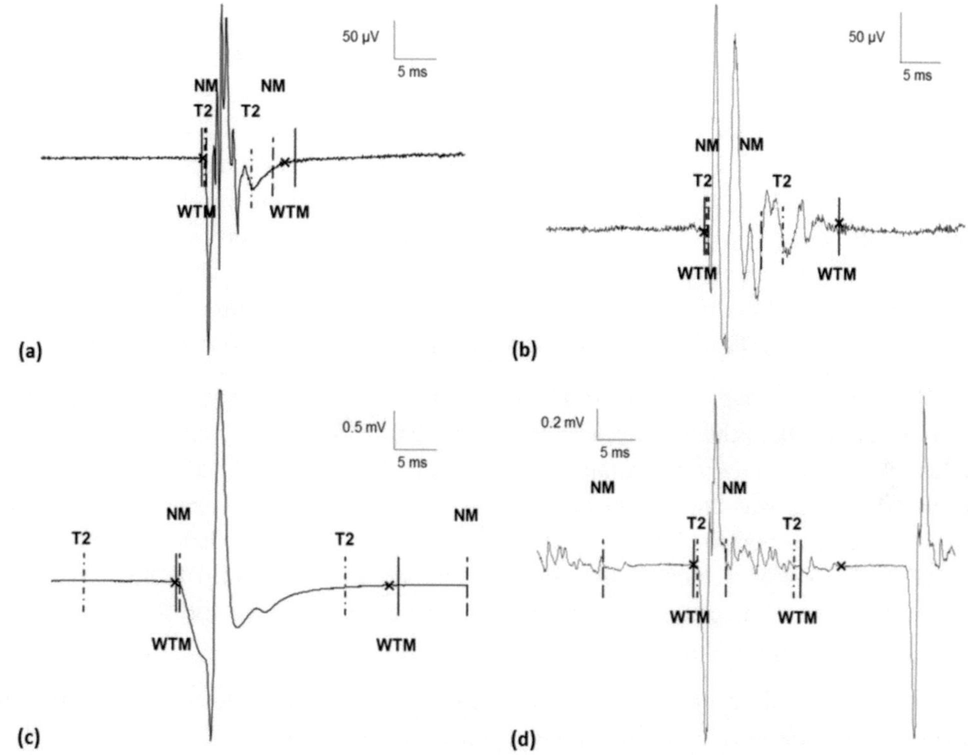


**Figure 10.** Performance of the CAMs with best results (T2 and NM) and the new duration method based on the wavelet transform (WTM) in pathological MUAPs: myopathic (a), subacute neurogenic (b), and chronic neurogenic MUAPs (c and d).

## 9. New techniques of automatic measurement of MUAP duration

The computational capacity of new computer systems enables the design and implementation of more complex algorithms for the automatic processing of the EMG recordings. Signal processing techniques such as the wavelet transform have been applied in the research and development of alternative automatic algorithms for measurement of MUAP duration.

The discrete wavelet transform (DWT) is a technique that simultaneously obtains a time and a scale representation of signals and has been successfully applied for detecting biological events [48]. This technique has provided promising results in the analysis of various electrophysiological signals such as blink reflex [49], EMG and electrocardiographic recordings [50-52], electroencephalographic signals for analysis of epileptic activity [53], and event-related potentials [54]. By regarding transformed EMG signals at a suitable scale in the DWT domain, it is possible to evade high frequency noise and low frequency BL fluctuations. Thus the DWT provides a useful way to detect the boundaries between the MUAP waveform and the BL, that is, for measuring MUAP duration.

A method based on the DWT was applied for measuring the MUAP duration [45, 55]. A schematic description of this method is given in Figure 11. The MUAP waveform consists of a set of peaks (Figure 11a) and the method makes use of the DWT with the non-orthogonal quadratic spline wavelet to detect not only the MUAP but also the start and end points of these peaks. The method selects two intermediate scales (one to find the start and another to find the end marker) from the DWT (Figure 11b) that represents the MUAP signal in terms of energy (thereby evading noise and BL fluctuation). In these DWT scales the peaks related to MUAP peaks are identified (Figure 11c) and amplitude and slope thresholds are used to determine MUAP start and end points (Figure. 11d). For finding MUAP start and end markers, this wavelet transform method (WTM) makes use of 10 parameters, which include the amplitude and slope thresholds. In the study, a genetic algorithm was applied to a sample of normal MUAPs in order to calculate the values of the WTM parameters [56].

This DWT-based automatic method was compared to other available algorithms and found to perform excellently, achieving accurate results for both normal and pathological MUAPs. Duration marker positions were significantly better than those of the other CAMs tested: the DWT-based method was the least biased and the most precise method as evidenced by the fact that it demonstrated the lowest mean and the lowest standard deviation of differences to the GSP. These improvements were observed with both normal and pathologic MUAPs, including myopathic, subacute and chronic neurogenic MUAPs, and also with fibrillation potentials [45, 55] (Figure 10).

The DWT-based method deals better with problems such as the presence of secondary MUAPs, BL fluctuations or high-frequency noise, performing equally well on signals recorded by various different commercial EMG hardware with varying amounts of technical noise. The rate of gross aberrant errors in start marker placement is low: 2.9, 0.8 or 0.0% for normal MUAPs, myopathic MUAPs and fibrillations, respectively. For the end marker, gross errors were more frequent: up to 27.6% for chronic neurogenic MUAPs, and around 10% for other kinds of pathologic MUAPs and for normal MUAPs. Although having less influence in the DWT-based method, the sources of error are the same as those for the other CAMs tested: long and high polyphasic waveforms (such as in chronic neurogenic MUAPs), the presence of consecutive peaks with low amplitude variation in initial or terminal parts (Figure 12a), and a low-sloped tail in the terminal part (Figure 12b). The latter is not detected by the DWT method because there is no corresponding maximum-minimum pair in the DWT.

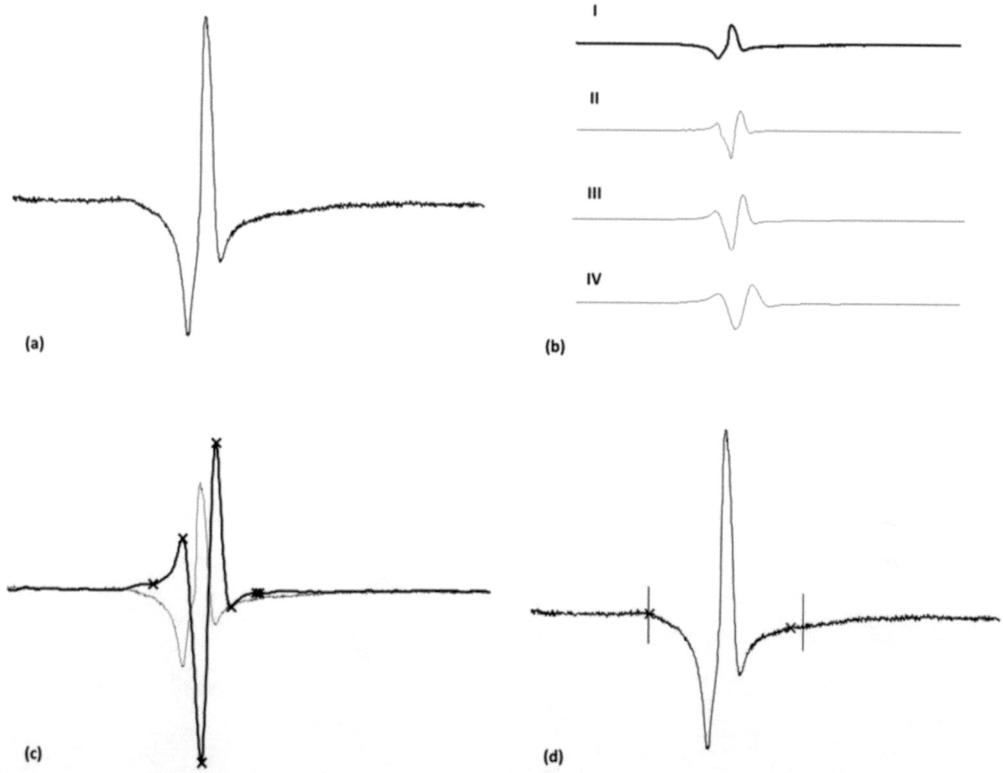


**Figure 11.** New method based on the DWT. (a) Original MUAP. (b) The MUAP (I) and the DWT at scales 4 (II), 5 (III) and 6 (IV). (c) MUAP and selected wavelet scale (thick continuous line) for finding start and end points. Maxima and minima related to the MUAP for the start and the end (thick crosses). (d) MUAP duration. Onset and offset (vertical lines) are shown and also the GSP (crosses) for this MUAP.

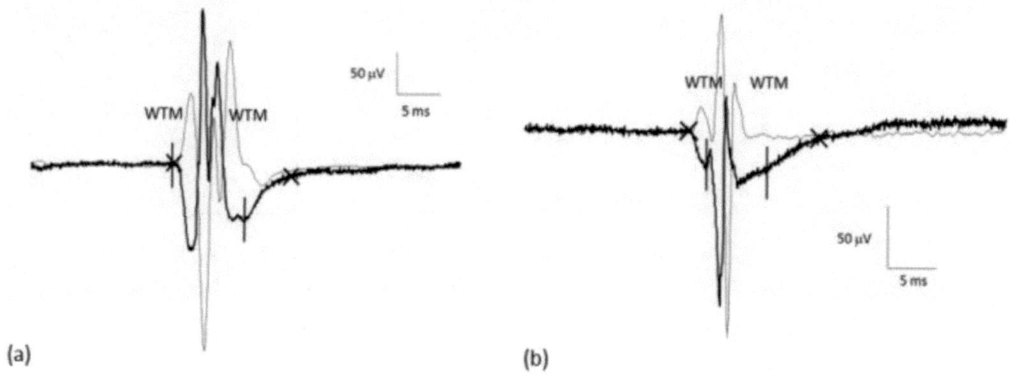


**Figure 12.** Errors in WTM start position in MUAPs with a small turn in their final (a) or initial part (b). Error in WTM in the end position in the low-slope tail of a MUAP in its terminal part (b). The waveform of the MUAPs (thick black line) and their selected scales of the DWT (thin grey line) are shown. GSP are in crosses.

DWT-based automatic duration marker positions were compared with the corresponding manual positions for a small set of repeatedly recorded MUAPs. While no significant differences were found for the start point, the dispersion of automatic endpoint placements was lower than the dispersion of the corresponding manual placements. This points at the possibility of reaching more consistent estimates of this parameter with automatic procedures than with manual measurements.

## 10. Conclusions and future perspectives

The measurement of MUAP duration is a matter of particular difficulty. Especially difficult is placement of a MUAP's endpoint marker, and this is reflected in the high degree of variability observed in manual measurements of MUAP duration. Neither is the accuracy of automatic measurement of MUAP duration good, and thus continuous supervision and frequent manual revision of duration marker position are necessary. (Figure 13). Such manual adjustments are time consuming and tedious and still do not guarantee accuracy.

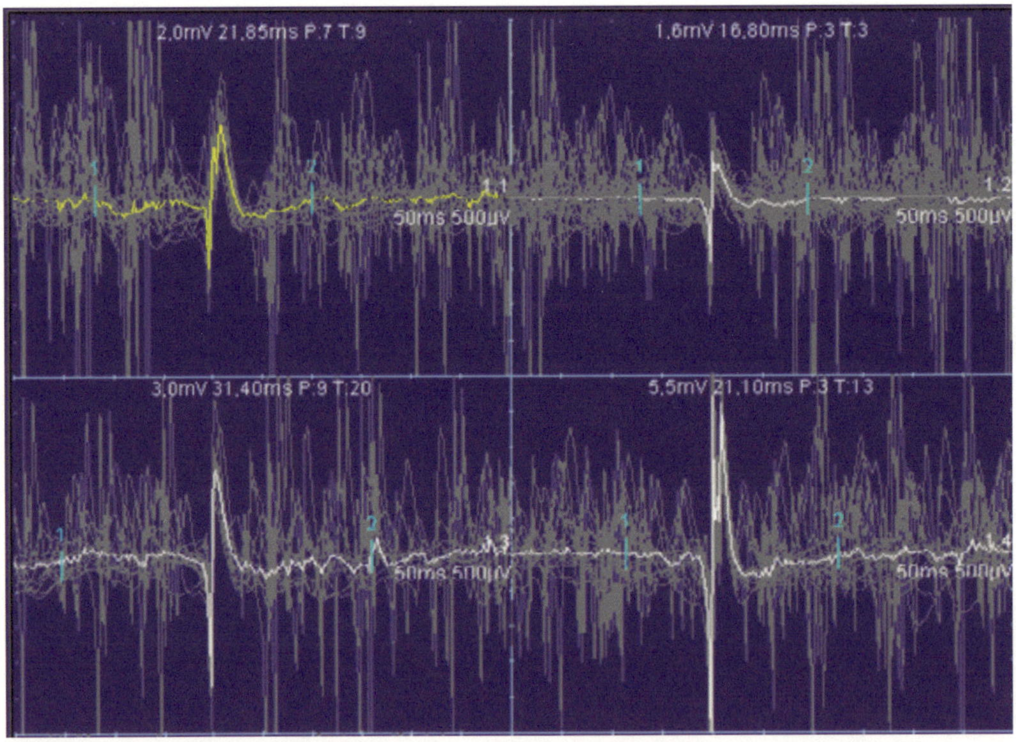


**Figure 13.** MUAPs automatically extracted by commercial equipment. MUAP durations are erroneously calculated and therefore manual corrections are needed.

Given the intrinsic difficulties, the measurement of MUAP duration has been described, quite correctly, as "an arbitrary task" [57]. However, the measurement of MUAP duration cannot be bypassed or avoided: not only does duration provide physiological information about the MU, it also delimits the MUAP waveform within which other MUAP parameters are measured. Thus, measurement of MUAP duration is an essential issue in EMG examinations, and it is of necessity the first task that must be accomplished before determination of other MUAP features.

Since we must have a measurement of MUAP duration, there is a strong requirement for a method which can provide "acceptable" estimations. By "acceptable" we recognize that there is not a unique true value of clinical duration. As has been discussed above, manual measurement does not ensure consistent estimates but there is reason to hope that an automatic method could be consistent enough. An automatic method might be considered good if it never makes gross misplacements, demonstrates low variability, works in real time and can deal with the relatively noisy signals found in daily clinical practice. An automatic method will show maximum repeatability because it will always give the same positions markers on re-analysis of a given MUAP input signal. If an effective automatic method suffers from any bias in marker positioning, it will be systematic and homogeneous in trend and magnitude, not arbitrary as occurs with subjective manual placements. Thus, the ideal method for attaining satisfactory consistency in MUAP duration measurement is an automatic method, which will overcome the inherent variability of human assessment.

The new, DWT-based computational strategy described above has demonstrated clear improvement in performance relative to conventional algorithms. There is, however, still significant room for betterment. More important than the results *per se* is the indication that some of the seemingly intractable difficulties in the management of bioelectrical recordings can be successfully overcome by new technologies of signal processing. The relevance of this conclusion extends beyond the area of EMG studies: the problems related to noise and variability in MU recording and measurement procedures are present in all the modalities of neurophysiologic studies and in Electromedicine in general. The measurement of MUAP duration is illustrative of the problematic nature of the analysis of bioelectric signals, but can be approached and managed with the latest signal processing techniques. Indeed, these techniques are being applied to other EMG features [58], such as the study of muscular fatigue [59], decomposition of surface EMG recordings [60, 61] and noise reduction for MUAPs extraction [62].

With respect to MUAP duration, further theoretical and empirical research is needed to develop automatic methods to provide robust and objective measurements, so that the MUAP duration measurement ceases to be an arbitrary task. Accurate and reliable automatic measurement of MUAP duration running on commercial equipment will serve to reduce the requirement for manual intervention in duration marker placement thereby helping the electromyographist. Together with multi-MUAP systems, automatic measurement methods could also contribute to a reduction in patient discomfort by shortening the examination time. Moreover, the availability of robust duration measurements would provide data of sufficient consistency and comparability for input into expert systems for diagnostic purposes, a natural goal of medical technology in the 21st Century.

## Author details

Ignacio Rodríguez-Carreño
*Universidad de Navarra, Department of Quantitative Methods in Economics, Pamplona, Spain*

Luis Gila-Useros
*Complejo Hospitalario de Navarra, Clinical Neurophysiology Service, Pamplona, Spain*

Armando Malanda-Trigueros
*Universidad Pública de Navarra, Department of Electrical and Electronic Engineering, Pamplona, Spain*

## 11. References

[1] Kimura J (2001). Electrodiagnosis in diseases of nerve and muscle: principles and practice. 3rd edition. New York: Oxford University Press.
[2] Dumitru D, Amato AA, Zwarts M. (2002). Electrodiagnostic medicine. 2nd edition. Hanley Belfus, Philadelphia,
[3] Stalberg E, Nandedkar S, Sanders DB, Falck B (1996). Quantitative motor unit potential analysis. J Clin Neurophysiol. 13: 401-422.
[4] Katz B (1966). Nerve, muscle, and synapse. McGraw-Hill, New York,.
[5] Feinstein B, Lindegard B, Nyman E, Wohlfart G (1955). Morphologic studies of motor units in normal human muscles. Acta Anat; 23: 127-142.
[6] Nandedkar S, Sanders D, Stalberg E (1985). Selectivity of electromyography recording techniques: a simulation study. Med Biol Eng Comp; 23: 536-540.
[7] Nandedkar S, Sanders D, Stalberg E, Andreassen S (1988). Simulation of concentric needle EMG motor unit action potentials. Muscle Nerve; 11: 151-159.
[8] Stalberg E, Trontelj J (1994). Single fiber electromyography in healthy and diseased muscle. 2nd edition. Raven Press, New York, 291 p.
[9] Nandedkar S, Barkhaus P, Sanders D, Stalberg E (1988). Analysis of the amplitude and area of the concentric needle EMG motor unit action potentials. Electroencephalogr Clin Neurophysiol; 69: 561-567.
[10] Sonoo M, Stalberg E (1993). The ability of PAUM parameters to discriminate between normal and neurogenic PAUMs in concentric EMG: analysis of the PAUM "thickness" and the proposal of "size index". Electroencephalogr Clin Neurophysiol; 89: 291-303.
[11] Stewart C, Nandedkar S, Massey J, Gilchrist J, Barkhaus P, Sanders D (1989). Evaluation of an automatic method of measuring features of motor unit action potentials. Muscle Nerve; 12: 141-148.
[12] Zalewska E, Hausmanowa-Petrusewicz I (1995). Evaluation of MUAP shape irregularity—a new concept of quantification. IEEE Trans Biomed Eng; 42: 616-620.
[13] Zalewska E, Rowinska-Marcinska K, Hausmanowa-Petrusevicz I (1998). Shape irregularity of motor unit potentials in some neuromuscular disorders. Muscle Nerve; 21: 1181-1187.

[14] Stalberg E, Sonoo M (1994). Assessment of variability in the shape of the motor unit action potential, the "jiggle," at consecutive discharges. Muscle Nerve; 17: 1135-1144.

[15] Campos C, Malanda A, Gila L, Segura V, Lasanta MI, Artieda J (2000). Quantification of jiggle in real electromyographic signals. Muscle Nerve; 23: 1022-1034.

[16] Stalberg E, Andreassen S, Falck B, Lang H, Rosenfalck A, Trojaborg W (1986). Quantitative analysis of individual motor unit potentials - a proposition for standardized terminology and criteria for measurement. J Clin Neurophysiol; 3: 313-348.

[17] Lang A, Tuomola H (1974). The time parameter of motor unit potentials recorded with multi-electrode and the summation technique. Electromyogr Clin Neurophysiol; 14: 513-525.

[18] Buchthal F, Guld C, Rosenfalck P (1954). Action potential parameters in normal muscle and their dependence on physical variables. Acta Physiol Scand; 32: 200.

[19] Thiele B, Boehle A (1978). Anzahl der Spike-Komponenten im Motor Unit Potential. EEG-EMG-Zeitung Elektroenzephogr Vervandte Geb;9:125-130

[20] Lang A, Partanen J (1976). "Satellite potentials" and the duration of potentials in normal, neuropathic and myopathic muscles. J Neurol Sci; 27: 513-524.

[21] Kosarov D, Gydikov A (1970). The influence of volume conduction on the shape of action potentials recorded by various types of needle electrodes in normal human muscles. Electromyogr Clin Neurophysiol; 333: 319-325.

[22] Chu J, Chan RC, Bruyninckx F (1986). Effects of the EMG amplifier settings on the motor unit action potential parameters recorded with concentric and monopolar needles. Electromyogr Clin Neurophysiol; 26: 627-639.

[23] Lang A, Vaahtoranta K (1973). The baseline, the time characteristics and the slow afterwaves of the motor unit potential. Electroencephalogr Clin Neurophysiol; 35: 387-394.

[24] Ma JA, Liveson DM (1992). Laboratory reference of clinical neurophysiology. F.A. Davis, Philadelphia.

[25] Buchthal F, Rosenfalck P (1955). Action potential parameters in different human muscles. Acta Psychiatr Scand; 30: 25-131.

[26] Bischoff C, Stalberg E, Falck B, Edebol Eeg-Olofsson K (1994). Reference values of motor unit action potentials obtained with multi-MUAP analysis. Muscle Nerve; 17: 842-851.

[27] Howard J, McGill K, Dorfman L (1988). Age effects on properties of motor unit action potentials: ADEMG analysis. Ann Neurol; 24: 207-213.

[28] Dorfman L, Robinson L (1997). AAEM Minimonograph 47: normative data in electrodiagnostic medicine. Muscle Nerve; 20: 4-14.

[29] Dumitru D, King JC (1999). Motor unit action potential duration and muscle lenght. Muscle Nerve; 22: 1188-1195.

[30] Dumitru D, King JC, Zwarts MJ (1999). Determinants of motor unit action potential duration. Clin Neurophysiol; 110: 1876-1882.

[31] Lateva Z, McGill K (1998). The physiological origin of the slow afterwave in muscle action potentials. Electroencephalogr Clin Neurophysiol; 109: 462-469.

[32] Bromberg MB, Smith AG, Bauerle J (1999). A comparison of two commercial quantitative electromyographic algorithms with manual analysis. Muscle Nerve; 22: 1244-1248.

[33] Pfeiffer G, Kunze K (1992). Turn and phase counts of individual motor unit potentials: correlation and reliability. Electroencephalogr Clin Neurophysiol; 85: 161-165.

[34] Stalberg E, Falck B, Sonoo M, Astrom M (1995). Multi-MUP EMG analysis—a two year experience with a quantitative method in daily routine. Electroencephalogr Clin Neurophysiol; 97: 145-154.

[35] Nandedkar S, Barkhaus P, Charles A (1995). Multi-motor unit action potential analysis (MMA). Muscle Nerve; 18: 1155-1166.

[36] Nirkko AC, Rösler KM, Hess CW (1995). Sensitivity and specificity of needle electromyography: a prospective study comparing automated interference pattern analysis with single motor unit potential analysis. Electroencephalogr Clin Neurophysiol; 97: 1-10.

[37] Takehara I, Chu J, Li TC, Schwartz I (2004). Reliability of quantitative motor unit action potential parameters. Muscle Nerve; 30: 111-113.

[38] Chu J, Takehara I, Li TC, Schwartz I (2003). Skill and selection bias has least influence on motor unit action potential firing rate/frequency. Electromyogr Clin Neurophysiol; 43: 387-392.

[39] Nandedkar S, Barkhaus P, Sanders D, Stalberg E (1988). Analysis of the amplitude and area of the concentric needle EMG motor unit action potentials. Electroencephalogr Clin Neurophysiol; 69: 561-567.

[40] Montgomery DC, Runger GC (1993). Gage capability and designed experiments. Part I: Basic methods. Quality Engineering; 6. pp. 115-135.

[41] Montgomery DC, Runger GC (1993). Gage capability and designed experiments. Part II: Experimental design models and variance component estimation. Quality Engineering; 6. pp 289-305.

[42] Rodríguez I, Gila L, Malanda A, Gurtubay I, Mallor F, Gómez S, Navallas J, Rodríguez J (2007). Motor unit action potential duration, I: variability of manual and automatic measurements. J Clin Neurophysiol; 24: 52-58.

[43] Automotive Industry Action Group (AIAG), (2002). Measurement systems analysis. 3rd edition.

[44] Takehara I, Chu J, Schwartz I, Aye HH (2004). Motor unit action potencial (MUAP) parameters affected by editing duration cursors. Electromyogr Clin Neurophysiol; 44: 265-269.

[45] Rodríguez I, Gila L, Malanda A, Gurtubay IG, Navallas J, Rodríguez J (2010). Application of a novel automatic duration method measurement based on the wavelet transform on pathological motor unit action potentials Clin Neurophysiol; 121: 1574-1583.

[46] Rodríguez I, Malanda A, Gila L, Navallas J, Rodríguez Falces J. Filter design for cancellation of baseline-fluctuation in needle EMG recordings (2006). Comput Methods Programs Biomed; 81: 79-93.

[47] Alvarez I, Rodríguez I, Gila L, Malanda A, Navallas J, Rodríguez J (2006). Influence of baseline fluctuation cancellation on automatic measurement of the motor unit action potential duration. Clin Neurophysiol; 117 (Suppl 1): S77.

[48] Akay M (1996). Detection and estimation methods of biomedical signals. Academic Press, New York,.

[49] Kumaran MS, Devasahayam SR, Sreedhar T (2000). Wavelet decomposition of the blik reflex R2 component enables improved discrimination of multiple sclerosis. Clin Neurophysiol; 111: 810-820.

[50] Fang J, Agarwall GC, Shahani BT (1999). Decomposition of multiunit electromyographic signals. IEEE Trans Biomed Eng; 46: 685-697.

[51] al-Fahoum AS, Howitt I (1999). Combined wavelet transformation and radial basis neural networks for classifying life-threatening cardiac arrhythmias. Med Biol Eng Comput; 37: 566-573.

[52] Cuiwei L, Chongxun Z, Changfen T (1995). Detection of ECG characteristic points using wavelet transforms. IEEE Trans Biomed Eng; 42: 21-28.

[53] Geva AB, Kerem DH (1998). Forecasting generalized epileptic seizures from the EEG signal by wavelet analysis and dynamic unsupervised fuzzy clustering. IEEE Trans Biomed Eng; 45: 1205-121.

[54] Gurtubay IG, Alegre M, Labarga A, Malanda A, Iriarte J, Artieda J (2001). Gamma band activity in an auditory oddball paradigm studied with the wavelet transform. Clin Neurophysiol; 112: 1219-1228.

[55] Rodríguez I, Gila L, Malanda A, Gurtubay I, Mallor F, Gómez S, Navallas J, Rodríguez J (2007). Motor unit action potential duration, II: a new automatic measurement method based on the wavelet transform. J Clin Neurophysiol; 24: 59-69.

[56] Goldberg DE (1989). Genetic algorithms in search, optimization and machine learning. Reading: Addison-Wesley,

[57] Sonoo M (2002). New attempts to quantify concentric needle electromyography. Muscle Nerve; Suppl 11: S98-S102.

[58] Raez MBI, Hussain MS, Mohd-Yasin F (2006). Techniques of EMG signal analysis: detection, processing, classification and applications. Biol Proced Online; 8: 11-35.

[59] Kumar DK, Pah ND, Bradley A (2003). Wavelet analysis of surface electromyography to determine muscle fatigue. IEEE Trans Neural Syst Rehabil Eng; 11: 400-406.

[60] Yamada R, Ushiba J, Tomita Y, Masakado Y (2003). Decomposition of electromyographic signal by principal component analysis of wavelet coefficient. IEEE EMBS Asian-Pacific Conference on Biomedical Engineering. Keihanna,: 118-119.

[61] Wimalaratna HS, Tooley MA, Churchill E, Preece AW, Morgan HM (2002). Quantitative surface EMG in the Diagnosis of neuromuscular disorders. Electromyogr Clin Neurophysiol; 42: 167-174.

[62] Ren X, Yan Z, Wang Z, Hu X (2006). Noise reduction based on ICA decomposition and wavelet transform for the extraction of motor unit action potentials. J Neurosci Methods; 158: 313-322.

Chapter 8

# The Neurocognitive Networks of the Executive Functions

Štefania Rusnáková and Ivan Rektor

Additional information is available at the end of the chapter

http://dx.doi.org/10.5772/51602

## 1. Introduction

Executive functions are associated with complex mental operations, such as planning, internal ordering, time perception, working memory, inhibition, self-monitoring, self-regulation, motor control, regulation of emotion, motivation (Norman & Shallice, 1986; Luu &Tucker; 2000).

## 2. Definition of particular components of the executive functions:

- **Planning**: organizational process of creating and maintaining a plan and the psychological process of thinking about the activities required to create a desired goal on some scale
- **Internal ordering:** A condition of logical or comprehensible arrangement among the separate elements of a group
- **Time perception:** timing of sensory information from multiple sensory streams is essential for many aspects of human perception and action
- **Working memory**: is a system for temporarily storing and managing the information required to carry out complex cognitive tasks such as learning, reasoning, and comprehension. Working memory is involved in the selection, initiation, and termination of information-processing functions such as encoding, storing, and retrieving data; that is the ability to hold information in mind and manipulate it.
- **Inhibition**: that is the ability to concentrate to execute task and to ignore distraction; function needed for goal-directed behaviour
- **Self-regulation:** self-directed action that serves to alter the probability of a subsequent response so as to alter the likelihood of a future consequence.
- **Self-monitoring:** self-discipline

- **Regulation of emotions:** self-regulation of emotions
- **Motivation:** refers to a process that elicits, controls, and sustains certain behaviours

Actions are executive if they involve the "when" or "whether" aspects of behaviour, whereas nonexecutive functions involve the "what" and "how."

The term *executive functions* seem to incorporate (Barkley, 1997):

- Volition, planning, and purposive, goal-directed, or intentional action
- Inhibition and resistance to distraction
- Problem-solving and strategy development, selection, and monitoring
- Flexible shifting of actions to meet task demands. Maintenance of persistence toward attaining a goal
- Self-awareness across time

## 3. Developmental aspects of executive functions

Mature cognition is characterized by abilities that include being able:

- to hold information in mind, including complicated representional structures to mentally manipulate that information, and to act on the basis of it
- to act on the basis of choice rather than impulse, exercising self-control by resisting inappropriate behaviors and responding appropriately
- to quickly and flexibly adapt behavior to changing situations

These abilities are referees to respectively as working memory, inhibition, and cognitive flexibility. Together they are key components of both "cognitive control" and "executive functions" (Davidson MC et al; 2006).

When studying executive functions, a developmental framework is helpful because these abilities mature at different rates over time. Some abilities peak in late childhood or adolescence while others progress into early adulthood. Furthermore, executive functioning development corresponds to the neurophysiological developments of the growing brain; as the processing capacity of the frontal lobes and other interconnected regions increases the core executive functions emerge (Lucca & Leventer 2008; Anderson 2002).

## 4. Childhood

Inhibitory control and working memory are among the earliest executive functions to appear, with initial signs observed in infants, 7 to 12-months old. Then in the preschool years, children display a spurt in performance on tasks of inhibition and working memory, usually between the ages of 3 to 5 years. Also during this time, cognitive flexibility, goal-directed behavior, and planning begin to develop (Lucca & Leventer 2008; Anderson 2002). Also between 8 and 12 months, infants are able to hold in mind for progressive longer period where a desired objects has been hidden, and are able to control their behavior so that they do not repeat a previously correct search that would not be wrong (Diamond

2006). Nevertheless, preschool children do not have fully mature executive functions and continue to make errors related to these emerging abilities - often not due to the absence of the abilities, but rather because they lack the awareness to know when and how to use particular strategies in particular contexts (Espy 2004). In the human brain, dendrites of pyramidal neurons in layer III of dorsolateral prefrontal cortex undergo their most dramatic expansion between the ages of $7^{1/2}$ and 12 months. Pyramidal neurons in dorsolateral prefrontal cortex have relatively short dendritic extents at $7^{1/2}$ months, but reach their full mature extent by 12 months (Koenderink, Ulyings and Mrzljiak; 1994). The level of glucose metabolism in in dorsolateral prefrontal cortex increases during this period as well, approximating adult levels by 1 year of age (Chugani, Phelps and Mazziotta, 1987). One particularly important developmental change during this period might be increased levels of dopamine in dorsolateral prefrontal cortex. Dopamine is important neurotransmitter in prefrontal cortex and reducing dopamine in prefrontal cortex impairs performance on executive function task (Brozoski, Brownm Resvold and Goldman, 1979; Diamond, 2001).

## 5. Preadolescence

Preadolescent children continue to exhibit certain growth spurts in executive functions. During preadolescence, children display major increases in verbal working memory, response inhibition, selective attention, goal-directed behavior and strategic planning (Brocki 2004; Anderson 2001; Klimkeit 2004). Between the ages of 8 to 10, cognitive flexibility in particular begins to match adult levels (Lucca 2003; Luciana 2002). However, similar to patterns in childhood development, executive functioning in preadolescents is limited because they do not reliably apply these executive functions across multiple contexts as a result of ongoing development of inhibitory control (de Lucca 2008).

## 6. Adolescence

During adolescence different brain systems become better integrated. At this time, youth implement executive functions, such as inhibitory control improve. Just as inhibitory control emerges in childhood and improves over time, planning and goal-directed behavior also demonstrate an extended time course with ongoing growth over adolescence. Likewise, functions such as attentional control, with a potential spurt at age 15, along with working memory, continue developing at this stage (Anderson et al, 2001).

## 7. Adulthood

The major change that occurs in the brain in adulthood is the constant myelination of neurons in the prefrontal cortex. At age 20-29, executive functioning skills are at their peak, which allows people of this age to participate in some of the most challenging mental tasks. These skills begin to decline in later adulthood. Working memory and spatial span are areas where decline is most readily noted (de Lucca et al, 2008).

## 8. The neurocognitive networks of the executive functions

Cognitive models typically describe executive functions as higher-level processes that exert control over elementary mental operations (Norman and Shallice, 1986; Luu and Tucker, 2002). A central position of the prefrontal cortex (PFC) and its cortical and sub-cortical connections in processing the executive functions have been suggested (Stuss and Benson, 1986; Badgaiyan, 2000). Ventromedial PFC is involved in decision-making processes, the dorsolateral portion has a role in working memory, planning and sequencing of behaviour. The caudal PFC is reported to be involved in attentional mechanism (Goldberg and Bruce, 1985). This theory was reviewed by Parkin (Parkin, 1998) who criticized the concept of the central position of the PFC in the executive functions. He suggested instead a pattern of extensive heterogenity with different executive tasks associated with different neural substrates. In fact, several studies have documented the diversity of executive functions and related anatomy (Godefroy, 2003).

Recent findings show that executive functions and cognition are associated with a lot of other structures.

## 9. Methods of neurocognitive network research

### 9.1. Cognitive ERP

Endogenous event-related potentials (ERPs) are thought to reflect the neurophysiologic correlates of cognitive processes. The P3 component of ERPs, which is a target detection response, has been one most studied. This long-latency waveform (300 milliseconds range) may represented various functions, such as closure of sensory analysis, cognitive closure of the recognition processing, the attentional and decisional processes and the update of working memory (Roesler et al, 1986; Verleger et al, 1994, 2005; Comerchero and Polich, 1999).

The main ERP components were identified by visual inspection and quantified by latency and amplitude measures. P3-like waves were identified in the 250-600 milliseconds latency range.

In our study (Rusnáková et al, 2011) the occurrence of the local generators of P3 like potentials, elicited by a noise-compatibility flanker test was used in order to study the processing of executive functions, particularly in the frontal and temporal cortices.

The test performed with arrows comprised a simpler congruent and a more difficult incongruent task. The two tasks activated the attention and several particular executive functions i.e. working memory, time perception, initiation and motor control of executed task. The incongruent task increased demand on executive functions, and beside the functions common for both tasks an inhibition of automatic responses, the reversal of incorrect response tendency, the internal ordering of the correct response and the initiation of the target-induced correct response was involved. In seven epilepsy surgery candidates (4 males and 3 females), ranging in age from 26 to 38 years, multi-contact depth electrodes were implanted in 590 cortical sites. We focused on local sources of P3-like potentials. Only the "phase reversal" and "steep voltage change" were considered to be generators of the studied potentials, because of their significance as the accepted signs of proximity to generating structure (Vaughan et al., 1986; Halgren et al., 1995a, b).

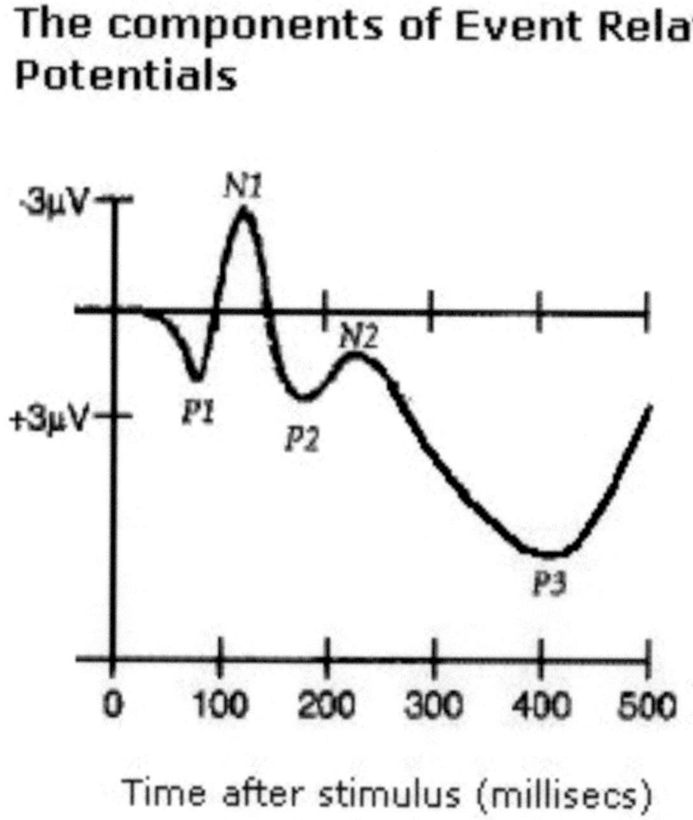


**Figure 1.**

In the two tasks, the P3 like potential sources were displayed in the mesial temporal structures; the lateral temporal neocortex; the anterior and posterior cingulate; the orbitofrontal cortex and dorsolateral prefrontal cortex. The P3 like potentials occurred more frequently with the incongruent than with congruent stimuli in all these areas. This more frequent occurrence of P3 sources elicited by the incongruent task appeared significant in temporal lateral neocortex and orbitofrontal cortex.

### 9.2. Event-related synchronization and desynchronization (ERD/S)

Event- related synchronization and desynchronization (ERD/S) represents a quantitative nonlinear EEG signal analysis method that enables to evaluate the changes of the background activity in any frequency ranges. These changes are related to an external or internal stimulus and are linked to the brain activation. It is widely used in the neuroscience research as a form of functional brain mapping. Especially the intracerebral recording data analysis have a big importance.

In a previous intracerebral depth electrodes study (Bočková et al., 2007) the neurocognitive network in the frontal and lateral temporal cortices was investigated by a visual-motor tasks of writing of single letters. The first task consisted of copying letters appearing on a monitor. In the second task, the patients were requested to write any other letter. The cognitive load of the second task was increased mainly by larger involvement of the executive functions. The task-related Event Related Desynchronization/Synchronization (ERD/ERS) of the alpha, beta and gamma rhythms was studied. The alpha and beta ERD/ERS linked specifically to the increased cognitive load was present in the PFC, the orbitofrontal cortex and surprisingly also the temporal neocortex. Particularly the TLC was activated by the increased cognitive load. It was suggested that the TLC together with frontal areas forms a cognitive network processing executive functions. The test used in Bočková's study consisted from an original and rather complex task, with involvement of several executive and non-executive processes. In consequence, the interpretation was rather complex. In order to confirm the suggested involvement of the TLC in the central executive we decided to perform the present study with a test that has been commonly used for studying executive functions

In conclusion, in Bočková et al. cognitive intracerebral studies was documented using ERD/S methodology the involvement of the lateral temporal neocortex in the neurocognitive network of executive functions.

## 9.3. Functional magnetic resonance (fMRI)

During the last decade occurred brisk development of the method of functional MRI which maps of regional changes of cerebral perfusion and indirectly assesses also the neuronal activation in the examined parts of the brain. It´s contribution to investigations of cognitive functions is not quite unequivocal so far. In the study of Brázdil et al. (2003) auditory "oddball" task examination was performed in 10 healthy volunteers using the method of "event-related" functional MRI (efMRI). The authors compared the assembled results with the results of previous efMRI and intracerebral ERP studies with the objective to evaluate the extent of agreement between areas with haemodynamically significantly different response to rare target stimuli and known intracerebral generator of the P3 potential. Both methods proved the activation of several areas in particular the parietal and frontal lobe (lobulus parietalis superior, inferior, gyrus supramarginalis, gyrus cinguli, of the lateral prefrontal cortex, gyrus temporalis superior and of the thalamus). Consistent with the assumed significant role of the neurocognitive network for directed attention in the course of detection of target stimuli in the majority of these structures a more marked haemodynamic response was observed on the right side. Against expectation in the presented experiment nor in any previous efMRI studies a significant haemodynamic response to target stimuli was not proved at the side of the most marked P3 generator in the amygdalohippocampal complex. Different results were also obtained on examination of further areas, e.g. rostral cingulum. Thus although the contribution of efMRI to recognition of the neuroanatomical correlate of mental processes is extremely high, it is unable to provide alone a complete map of activated cerebral areas in the course of cognitive operations. The reason is most probably the inability to reflect fully transient short-term mentary method and it´s results must be evaluated with maximum caution (Brázdil et al; 2003).

## 10. Conclusion

Intracranial and neuroimaging studies demonstrated a widespread distribution of cognitive ERPs in multiple cortical and subcortical regions in the human brain. The participation of the frontal, temporal and parietal cortices, in addition to the cingulate and mesial temporal regions, the basal ganglia and thalamus, has been shown with visual, auditory and somatosensory stimuli (Halgren et al., 1995 a,b, 1998; Clarke et al., 1999, 2003; Smith et al., 1990; Baudena et al., 1995; Lamarche et al., 1995; Brázdil et al., 1999, 2003; Rektor et al., 2001 a,b, 2004, 2007; Bočkova et al 2007; Rusnáková et al. 2011).

Based on other studies (Baláž et al, 2008; Rektor et al, 2009; Bočková et al.), even subthalamic nucleus (STN) is a part of widespread neurocognitive network. Cognitive activities in the STN could be explained by existence of hyperdirect cortico-STN pathway. Certain effect of deep brain stimulation (DBS) on cognitive performance is possibly caused by a direct influence on ´cognitive´ parts of STN (Rektor et al, 2009).

In conclusion, reviewed studies, confirm theory of widespread and complex neurocognitive network of the executive functions.

## Abbreviations

EEG: electroencephalography
ERD/ERS: Event Related Desynchronization/Synchronization
ERPs: event-related potentials
fMRI: functional magnetic resonance imaging
efMRI: event-related functional magnetic resonance imaging
FT: Flanker test

## Author details

Štefania Rusnáková *
*Department of Neurology, Masaryk University, St. Anne´s Hospital, Brno, Czech Republic*

*Clinic of Child Neurology, University Hospital Brno, Czech Republic*

Ivan Rektor
*Department of Neurology, Masaryk University, St. Anne´s Hospital, Brno, Czech Republic*

* Corresponding Author

## Acknowledgement

This study was supported by a grant from PharmAround project number CZ.1.07/2.4.00/17.0034.

## 11. References

Anderson VA, Anderson P, Northan E, Jacobs R, Catroppa C. Development of executive functions through late childhood and adolescence in an Australian sample". *Developmental Neuropsychology* 2001; 20 (1): 385–406.

Anderson PJ: Assessment and development of executive functioning (EF) in childhood". *Child Neuropsychology* 8 (2): 71–82; 2002.

Badgaiyan RD. Executive control, willed actions, and nonconscious processing. *Hum Brain Mapp* 2000; 9:38-41.

Baláž M, Rektor I, Pulkrábek J. Participation of the subthalamic nucleus in executive functions: An intracerebral recording study. Movement disorders 2008; 23:553-557.

Barkley, R. A. Behavioral inhibition, sustained attention, and executive functions: constructing a unifying theory of ADHD. Psychol. Bull., 1997 b, 121: 65±94.

Baudena P, Halgren E, Heit G, Clarke JM. Intracerebral potentials to rare target and distractor auditory and visual stimuli III. Frontal cortex. *Electroencephalogr Clin Neurophysiol* 1995; 94:251-264.

Bockova M, Chladek J, Jurak P, Halamek J, Rektor I. Executive functions processed in the frontal and lateral temporal cortices: intracerebral study. *Clin Neurophysiol* 2007; 118:2625-2636.

Brazdil M, Rektor I, Dufek M, Daniel P, Jurak P, Kuba R. The role of frontal and temporal lobes in visual discrimination task- depth ERP studies. *Neurophysiol Clin* 1999; 29: 339-350.

Brazdil M, Rektor I, Daniel P, Dufek M, Jurak P. Intracerebral event-related potentials to subthreshold target stimuli. *Clin Neurophysiol* 2001; 112:650-661.

Brázdil M, Dobšík M, Pažourková M, Krupa P, Rektor I.: Importance of Functional MRI for Evaluation of Cognitive Processes in the Human brain. Localization of neuronal population activated by „oddball" task. *Československá neurologie a neurochirurgie 60/99, 2003, No.1, 20-30.*

Brocki KC Bohlin G. Executive functions in children aged 6 to 13: A dimensional and developmental study;". *Developmental Neuropsychology 2004; 26 (2): 571–593.*

Brozoski TJ, Brown RM, Rosvold HE, Goldman PS. Cognitive deficit caused by regional depletion of dopamine in prefrontal cortex of rheus monkey. *Science, 1979, 205, 929-932.*

Bruce CJ, Goldberg ME. Primate frontal eye fields. I. Single neurons discharging before saccades. *J Neurophysiol* 1985;53:603-635.

Chugani HT, Phebs ME, Mazziotta JC. Positron emission tomography study of human brain functional development. *Annals of neurology, 1987, 22, 487-497.*

Comerchero MD, Polich J. P3a and P3b from typical auditory and visual stimuli. *Clin Neurophysiol* 1999;110:24-30.

De Luca CR, Leventer RJ: Developmental trajectories of executive functions across the lifespan". In Anderson V, Jacobs R, Anderson PJ. *Executive functions and the frontal lobes: A lifespan perspective*. New York: Taylor & Francis 2008; pp. 3–21.

De Luca CR, Wood SJ, Anderson V, Buchanan JA, Proffitt T, Mahoney K, Panteli C. Normative data from the CANTAB I: Development of executive function over the lifespan. *Journal of Clinical and Experimental Neuropsychology* 2003; 25 (2): 242–254.

Espy KA: Using developmental, cognitive, and neuroscience approaches to understand executive functions in preschool children". *Developmental Neuropsychology* 26 (1): 379–384; 2004.

Godefroy O. Frontal syndrome and disorders of executive functions. *Journal of Neurology* 2003; 1:1-6.

Halgren E, Baudena P, Clarke JM, et al. Intracerebral potentials to rare target and distractor auditory and visual stimuli I. Superior temporal plane and parietal lobe. *Electroencephalogr Clin Neurophysiol* 1995a; 94:191-220.

Halgren E, Baudena P, Clarke JM., et al. Intracerebral potentials to rare target and distractor auditory and visual stimuli. II. Medial, lateral and posterior temporal lobe. *Electroencephalogr Clin Neurophysiol* 1995b; 94:229-250.

Halgren E, Marinkovic K, Chauvel P. Generators of the late cognitive potentials in auditory and visual oddball tasks. *Electroencephalogr Clin Neurophysiol* 1998; 106,156-164.

Klimkeit EI, Mattingley JB, Sheppard DM, Farrow M, Bradshaw JL. Examining the development of attention and executive functions in children with a novel paradigm". *Child Neuropsychology* 2004; 10 (3): 201–211.

Koederink MJT, Ulyings HBM, Mrzljiak L. Postnatal maturation of the layer III pyramidal neurons in the human prefrontal cortex: A quantitative Golgi analysis. Brain research, 1994, 653, 173-182.

Luciana M, Nelson CA. Assessment of neuropsychological function through use of the Cambridge Neuropsychological Testing Automated Battery: Performance in 4- to 12-year old children. *Developmental Neuropsychology* 2002; 22(3): 595–624.

Luu P, Flaisch T, Tucker DM. Medial Frontal Cortex in Action Monitoring. *J Neurosci*, 2000, 20:464-469.

Davidson MC, Amso D, Anderson LC, Diamond A. Development of cognitive control and executive functions from 4 to 13 years: Evidence from manipulations of memory, inhibition, and task switching. *Neuropsychologia 2006; 44, 2037-2078*

Parkin AJ. The central executive does not exist. *J Int Neuropsychol Soc* 1998◎4:518-522.

Rektor I, Kanovsky P, Bares M, Louvel J, Lamarche M. Event-related potentials, CNV, readiness potential, and movement accompanying potential recorded from posterior thalamus in human subjects. A SEEG study. *Neurophysiol Clin* 2001a◎31:253-261.

Rektor I, Bares M, Kanovsky P, Kukleta M. Intracerebral recording of readiness potential induced by a complex motor task. *Mov Disord* 2001b 16:698-704.

Rektor I, Bares M, Kanovsky P. Cognitive potentials in the basal ganglia-frontocortical circuits. An intracerebral recording study. *Exp Brain Res* 2004 158:289-301.

Rektor I, Brazdil M, Nestrasil I, Bares M, Daniel P. Modifications of cognitive and motor tasks affect the occurrence of event-related potentials in the human cortex. *Eur J Neurosci* 2007, 26:1371-1380.

Rektor I, Baláž M, Bočková M. Cognitive activities in the subthalamic nukleus. Invasive studies. Parkinsonism and related disorders 2009; S82-S86.

Rosler F, Sutton S, Johnson R, et al. Endogenous ERP components and cognitive constructs. A review. Electroencephalogr Clin Neurophysiol Suppl 1986; 38:51-92.

Rusnáková Š, Daniel P, Chládek J, Jurák P, Rektor I. The Executive Functions in Frontal and Temporal Lobes: A Flanker Task Intracerebral Recording Study. Journal of Clinical Neurophysiology, Volume 28 - Issue 1 - pp 30-35; 2011.

Smith ME, Halgren E, Sokolik M, et al. The intracranial topography of the P3 event-related potential elicited during auditory oddball. *Electroencephalogr Clin Neurophysiol* 1990; 76: 235-248.

Verleger R, Heide W, Butt C, Kompf D. Reduction of P3b in patients with temporo-parietal lesions. Brain Res Cogn Brain Res 1994◎2:103-116.

Verleger R, Gorgen S, Jaskowski P. An ERP indicator of processing relevant gestalts in masked priming. Psychophysiology 2005◎ 42:677-690.

Chapter 9

# Mild Cognitive Impairment and Quantitative EEG Markers: Degenerative Versus Vascular Brain Damage

D. V. Moretti, G. B. Frisoni, G. Binetti and O. Zanetti

Additional information is available at the end of the chapter

http://dx.doi.org/10.5772/47881

## 1. Introduction

We evaluated the changes induced by cerebrovascular damage (CVD and ) and amigdalo-hippocampal atrophy (AHC) on brain rhythmicity as revelaled by scalp electroencephalography (EEG) in a cohort of subjects with mild cognitive impairment (MCI).

All MCI subjects (Mini-Mental State Examination [MMSE] mean score 26.6). All subjects underwent EEG recording and magnetic resonance imaging (MRI). EEGs were recorded at rest. Relative power was separately computed for delta, theta, alpha1, alpha2, and alpha3 frequency bands.

In the spectral bandpower the severity of cerebrovascular damage (CVD) was associated with increased delta power and decreased alpha2 power. No association of vascular damage was observed with alpha3 power. Moreover, the theta/alpha 1 ratio could be a reliable index for the estimation of the individual extent of CV damage. On the other side, the group with moderate hippocampal atrophy showed the highest increase of alpha2 and alpha3 power. Moreover, when the amygdalar and hippocampal volume (AHC) are separately considered, within AHC, the increase of theta/gamma ratio is best associated with amygdalar atrophy whereas alpha3/alpha2 ratio is best associated with hippocampal atrophy.

CVD and AHC are associated with specific EEG markers. So far, these EEG markers could have a prospective value in differential diagnosis between vascular and degenerative MCI. Moreover, EEG markers could be expression of different global network pathological changes, better explaining MCI state.

Mild cognitive impairment (MCI) is a clinical state intermediate between elderly normal cognition and dementia which affects a significant amount of the elderly population, featuring memory complaints and cognitive impairment on neuropsychological testing, but no dementia (Flicker et al., 1991; Petersen et al., 1995, 2001).

The hippocampus is one of the first and most affected brain regions impacted by both Alzheimer's disease and mild cognitive impairment (MCI; Arnold et al., 1991; Bobinski et al., 1995; Price and Morris, 1999; Schonheit et al., 2004; Bennett et al., 2005, Frisoni et al., 2009). In mild-to-moderate Alzheimer's disease patients, it has been shown that hippocampal volumes are 27% smaller than in normal elderly controls (Callen et al., 2001; Du et al., 2001), whereas patients with MCI show a volume reduction of 11% (Du et al., 2001). So far, from a neuropathological point of view, the progression of disease from early or very early MCI to later stages seems to follow a linear course. Nevertheless, there is some evidence from functional (Gold et al., 2000; Della Maggiore et al., 2002; Hamalaainen et al., 2006) and biochemical studies (Lavenex and Amaral, 2000) that the process of conversion from non-demented to clinically-evident demented state is not so linear. Recent fMRI studies have suggested increased medial temporal lobe (MTL) activations in MCI subjects vs controls, during the performance of memory tasks (Dickerson et al., 2004, 2005). Nonetheless, fMRI findings in MCI are discrepant, as MTL hypoactivation similar to that seen in AD patients (Pariente et al., 2005) has also been reported (Machulda et al., 2003). Recent postmortem data from subjects – who had been prospectively followed and clinically characterized up to immediately before their death – indicate that hippocampal choline acetyltransferase levels are reduced in Alzheimer's dementia, but in fact they are upregulated in MCI (Lavenex and Amaral, 2000), presumably because of reactive upregulations of the enzyme activity in the unaffected hippocampal cholinergic axons. Previous EEG studies (Jelic et al. 2000, 1996; Ferreri et al., 2003,Pijnenburg et al., 2004; Jiang et al., 2005, 2006, Zheng et al., 2007) have shown a decrease – ranging from 8 to 10.5 Hz (low alpha) – of the alpha frequency power band in MCI subjects, when compared to normal elderly controls (Zappoli et al., 1995; Huang et al., 2000; Jelic et al., 2000; Koenig et al., 2005; Babiloni et al., 2006). However, a recent study has shown an increase – ranging from 10.5 to 13 Hz (high alpha) – of the alpha frequency power band, on the occipital region in MCI subjects, when compared to normal elderly and AD patients (Babiloni et al., 2006). These somewhat contradictory findings may be explained by the possibility that MCI subjects have different patterns of plastic organization during the disease, and that the activation (or hypoactivation) of different cerebral areas is based on various degrees of hippocampal atrophy. If this hypothesis is true, then EEG changes of rhythmicity have to occur non-proportionally to the hippocampal atrophy, as previously demonstrated in a study of auditory evoked potentials (Golob et al, 2007).

In a recent study (Moretti et al., 2007a), the results confirm the hypothesis that the relationship between hippocampal volume and EEG rhythmicity is not proportional to the hippocampal atrophy, as revealed by the analyses of both the relative band powers and the individual alpha markers. Such a pattern seems to emerge because, rather than a classification based on clinical parameters, discrete hippocampal volume differences (about 1 $cm^3$) are analyzed. Indeed, the group with moderate hippocampal atrophy showed the highest increase in the theta power on frontal regions, and of the alpha2 and alpha3 powers on frontal and temporo-parietal areas.

Recently, two specific EEG markers, theta/gamma and alpha3/alpha2 frequency ratio have been reliable associated to the atrophy of amygdalo-hippocampal complex (Moretti et al.

2008), as well as with memory deficits, that are a major risk for the development of AD in MCI subjects (Moretti et al., 2009). Based on the tertiles values of decreasing AHC volume, three groups of AHC growing atrophy were obtained. AHC atrophy is associated with memory deficits as well as with increase of theta/gamma and alpha3/alpha2 ratio. Moreover, when the amygdalar and hippocampal volume are separately considered, within AHC, the increase of theta/gamma ratio is best associated with amygdalar atrophy whereas alpha3/alpha2 ratio is best associated with hippocampal atrophy.

The role of cerebrovascular (CV) disease and ischemic brain damage in cognitive decline remains controversial. Although not all patients with mild cognitive impairment due to CV damage develop a clinically defined dementia, all such patients are at risk and could develop dementia in the 5 years following the detection of cognitive decline. Cognitive impairment due to subcortical CV damages is thought to be caused by focal or multifocal lesions involving strategic brain areas. These lesions in basal ganglia, thalamus or connecting white matter induce interruption of thalamocortical and striatocortical pathways. As a consequence, deafferentation of frontal and limbic cortical structures is produced. The pattern of cognitive impairment is consistent with models of impaired cortical and subcortical neuronal pathways (Kramer et al., 2002). Even when CV pathology appears to be the main underlying process, the effects of the damaged brain parenchyma are variable and, therefore, the clinical, radiological and pathological appearances may be heterogeneous. A neurophysiological approach could be helpful in differentiating structural from functional CV damage (Moretti et al., 2007b). The quantitative analysis of electroencephalographic (EEG) rhythms in resting subjects is a low-cost but still powerful approach to the study of elderly subjects in normal aging, MCI and dementia.

## 2. Materials and methods

### 2.1. Subjects

#### *2.1.1. Cerebrovascular impairment*

For the present study, 99 subjects with MCI were recruited. All experimental protocols had been approved by the local Ethics Committee. Informed consent was obtained from all participants or their caregivers, according to the Code of Ethics of the World Medical Association (Declaration of Helsinki). Table 1 shows the main features of this group.

| | GROUP 1 | GROUP 2 | GROUP 3 | GROUP 4 |
|---|---|---|---|---|
| SUBJECTS (F/M) | 27 (18/9) | 41 (31/10) | 19 (10/9) | 12 (9/3) |
| AGE | 70.1 (±1.7) | 69.9 (±1.1) | 69.7 (±1.9) | 70.5 (±2.4) |
| EDUCATION | 7.1 (±0.7) | 7 (±0.6) | 7 (±0.9) | 10 (±1.6) |
| MMSE | 26.7 (±0.4) | 26.5 (±0.4) | 27 (±0.4) | 26.1 (±0.7) |
| ARWMC scale | 0 | 1-5 | 6-10 | 11-15 |

Group 1, no vascular damage; group 2, mild vascular damage; group 3 moderate vascular damage; group 4, severe vascular damage.

**Table 1.** Mean values ± standard error of demographic characteristics, neuropsychological and ARWMC scores of the MCI subgroups. F/m, female/male. Age and education are expressed in years

## 2.2. Degenerative impairment

### *2.2.1. Subjects*

For the present study, 79 subjects with MCI were recruited from the memory Clinic of the Scientific Institute for Research and Care (IRCCS) of Alzheimer's and psychiatric diseases 'Fatebenefratelli' in Brescia, Italy. All experimental protocols had been approved by the local Ethics Committee. Informed consent was obtained from all participants or their caregivers, according to the Code of Ethics of the World Medical Association (Declaration of Helsinki). Table 2 shows the main characteristic of the group.

| | GROUP 1 | GROUP 2 | GROUP 3 | GROUP 4 |
|---|---|---|---|---|
| t/a1 | 0,7 (±0.05) | 0,77 (±0.05) | 1,17 (±0.05) | 1,39 (±0.14) |
| a1/a2 | 0,46 (±0.03) | 0,5 (±0.03) | 0,53 (±0.05) | 0,47 (±0.04) |
| a2/a3 | 1,27 (±0.12) | 1,16 (±0.1) | 0,85 (±0.05) | 0,79 (±0.07) |

Group 1, no vascular damage; group 2, mild vascular damage; group 3 moderate vascular damage; group 4, severe vascular damage.

**Table 2.** Mean values ± standard error of theta/alpha1, alpha1/alpha2, alpha2/alpha3 ratios in the MCI subgroups.

## 2.3. Shared procedures

### *2.3.1. EEG recordings*

All recordings were obtained in the morning with subjects resting comfortably. Vigilance was continuously monitored in order to avoid drowsiness.

The EEG activity was recorded continuously from 19 sites by using electrodes set in an elastic cap (Electro-Cap International, Inc.) and positioned according to the 10-20 International system (Fp1, Fp2, F7, F3, Fz, F4, F8, T3, C3, Cz, C4, T4, T5, P3, Pz, P4, T6, O1, O2). The ground electrode was placed in front of Fz. The left and right mastoids served as reference for all electrodes. The recordings were used off-line to re-reference the scalp recordings to the common average. Data were recorded with a band-pass filter of 0.3-70 Hz, and digitized at a sampling rate of 250 Hz (BrainAmp, BrainProducts, Germany). Electrodes-skin impedance was set below 5 kW. Horizontal and vertical eye movements were detected by recording the electrooculogram (EOG). The recording lasted 5 minutes, with subjects with closed eyes. Longer recordings would have reduced the variability of the data, but they would also have increased the possibility of slowing of EEG oscillations due to reduced vigilance and arousal. EEG data were then analyzed and fragmented off-line in consecutive epochs of 2 seconds, with a frequency resolution of 0.5 Hz. The average number of epochs analyzed was 140 ranging from 130 to150. The EEG epochs with ocular, muscular and other types of artifacts were discarded.

### 2.3.2. *Analysis of individual frequency bands*

A digital FFT-based power spectrum analysis (Welch technique, Hanning windowing function, no phase shift) computed – ranging from 2 to 45 Hz – the power density of EEG rhythms with a 0.5 Hz frequency resolution. Methods are exposed in detail elsewhere (Moretti et al., 2004, 2007a,b]. Briefly, two anchor frequencies were selected according to literature guidelines (Klimesch et al., 1999), that is, the theta/alpha transition frequency (TF) and the individual alpha frequency (IAF) peak. Based on TF and IAF, we estimated the following frequency band range for each subject: delta, theta, low alpha band (alpha1 and alpha2), and high alpha band (alpha3). Moreover, individual beta and gamma frequencies were computed. Three frequency peaks were detected in the frequency range from the individual alpha 3 frequency band and 45 Hz. These peaks were named beta1 peak (IBF 1), beta2 peak (IBF 2) and gamma peak (IGF). Based on peaks, the frequency ranges were determined. Beta1 ranges from alpha 3 to the lower spectral power value between beta1 and beta2 peak; beta2 frequency ranges from beta 1 to the lower spectral power value between beta2 and gamma peak; gamma frequency ranges from beta 2 to 45 Hz, which is the end of the range considered. The mean frequency range computed in MCI subjects considered as a whole are: delta 2.9-4.9 Hz; theta 4.9-6.9 Hz; alpha1 6.9-8.9 Hz; alpha2 8.9-10.9 Hz; alpha3 10.9-12-9 Hz; beta1 12,9-19,2 Hz; beta2 19.2-32.4; gamma 32.4-45. In the frequency bands determined in this way, the relative power spectra for each subject were computed. The relative power density for each frequency band was computed as the ratio between the absolute power and the mean power spectra from 2 to 45 Hz. Th9 relative band power at each band was defined as the mean of the relative band power for each frequency bin within that band. Finally, the theta/gamma and alpha3/alpha2 relative power ratio were computed and analyzed. The analysis of other frequencies was not in the scope of this study.

### 2.3.3. *Diagnostic criteria*

In this study we enrolled subjects afferents to the scientific institute of research and cure Fatebenefratelli in Brescia, Italy. Patients were taken from a prospective project on clinical progression of MCI. The project was aimed to study the natural history of non demented persons with apparently primary cognitive deficits, not caused by psychic (anxiety, depression, etc.) or physical (uncontrolled heart disease, uncontrolled diabetes, etc.) conditions. Patients were rated with a series of standardized diagnostic tests, including the Mini-Mental State Examination (MMSE; Folstein et al., 1975), the Clinical Dementia Rating Scale (CDRS; Hughes et al., 1982), the Hachinski Ischemic Scale (HIS; Rosen et al., 1980), and the Instrumental and Basic Activities of Daily Living (IADL, BADL, Lawton and Brodie, 1969). In addition, patients were subjected to diagnostic neuroimaging procedures (magnetic resonance imaging, MRI) and laboratory blood analysis to rule out other causes of cognitive impairment.

The present inclusion and exclusion criteria for MCI were based on previous seminal studies (Albert et al., 1991; Petersen et al., 1995, 1997, 2001; Portet et al., 2006; Geroldi et al., 2006). Inclusion criteria in the study were all of the following: (i) complaint by the patient or report by a relative or the general practitioner of memory or other cognitive disturbances; (ii) mini mental state examination (MMSE; Folstein et al., 1975) score of 24 to 27/30 or MMSE of 28 and higher plus low performance (score of 2/6 or higher) on the clock drawing test (Shulman, 2000); (iii) sparing of instrumental and basic activities of daily living or functional impairment stably due to causes other than cognitive impairment, such as physical impairments, sensory loss, gait or balance disturbances, etc. Exclusion criteria were any one of the following: (i) age of 90 years and older; (ii) history of depression or psychosis of juvenile onset; (iii) history or neurological signs of major stroke; (iv) other psychiatric diseases, epilepsy, drug addiction, alcohol dependence; (v) use of psychoactive drugs including acetylcholinesterase inhibitors or other drugs enhancing brain cognitive functions; and (vi) current or previous uncontrolled or complicated systemic diseases (including diabetes mellitus) or traumatic brain injuries.

All patients underwent: (i) semi-structured interview with the patient and – whenever possible – with another informant (usually the patient's spouse or a child) by a geriatrician or neurologist; (ii) physical and neurological examinations; (iii) performance-based tests of physical function, gait and balance; (iv) neuropsychological assessment evaluating verbal and non-verbal memory, attention and executive functions (Trail Making Test B-A; Clock Drawing Test; Amodio et al., 2000; Shulman, 2000), abstract thinking (Raven matrices; Basso et al., 1987), frontal functions (Inverted Motor Learning; Spinnler and Tognoni, 1987); language (Phonological and Semantic fluency; Token test; Carlesimo et al., 1996), and apraxia and visuo-constructional abilities (Rey figure copy; Caffarra et al., 2002); (v) assessment of depressive symptoms with the Center for Epidemiologic Studies Depression Scale (CES-D; Radloff, 1977). Given the aim of the study to evaluate the impact of vascular damage on EEG rhythms, in this study we did not consider the clinical subtype of MCI, i.e. amnesic, non amnesic or multiple domain.

## 2.4. Magnetic resonance imaging (MRI) and CV damage evaluation

Magnetic Resonance (MR) images were acquired using a 1.0 Tesla Philips Gyroscan. Axial T2 weighted, proton density (DP) and fluid attenuated inversion recovery (FLAIR) images were acquired with the following acquisition parameters: TR = 2000 ms, TE = 8.8/110 ms, flip angle = 90°, field of view = 230 mm, acquisition matrix 256x256, slice thickness 5 mm for T2/DP sequences and TR = 5000 ms, TE = 100 ms, flip angle = 90°, field of view = 230 mm, acquisition matrix 256x256, slice thickness 5 mm for FLAIR images.

Subcortical cerebrovascular disease (sCVD) was assessed using the rating scale for age-related white matter changes (ARWMC) on T2-weighted and FLAIR MR images. White matter changes (WMC) was rated by a single observer (R.R.) in the right and left hemispheres separately in frontal, parieto-occipital, temporal, infratentorial areas and basal ganglia on a 4 point scale. The observer of white matter changes was blind to the clinical information of the subjects. Subscores of 0, 1, 2, and 3 were assigned in frontal, parieto-occipital, temporal, infratentorial areas for: no WMC, focal lesions, beginning confluence of lesions, and diffuse involvement of the entire region, respectively. Subscores of 0, 1, 2, and 3 were assigned in basal ganglia for: no WMC, 1 focal lesion, more than 1 focal lesion and confluent lesions, respectively. Total score was the sum of subscores for each area in the left and right hemisphere, ranging from 0 to 30. As regards the ARWMC scale, the interrater reliability, as calculated with weighted k value, was 0.67, indicative of moderate agreement (Wahlund et al., 2001). We assessed test-retest reliability on a random sample of 20 subjects. The intraclass correlation coefficient was 0.98, values above 0.80 being considered indicative of good agreement.

Based on increasing subcortical CV damage, the 99 MCI subjects were subsequently divided in 4 sub-groups along the range between the minimum and maximum ARWMC score (respectively 0 and 15). In order to have the higher sensibility to the CV damage, the first group was composed by subjects with score = 0. The other groups were composed according to equal range ARWMC scores. As a consequence, we obtained the following groups: group 1 (G1) no vascular damage, CV score 0; group 1 (G2), mild vascular damage, CV score 1-5; group 3 (G3), moderate vascular damage, CV score 6-10; group 1 (G4), severe vascular damage, CV score 11-15.

Table 1 reports the mean values of demographic and clinical characteristics of the 4 subgroups.

## 2.5. Statistical analysis

Preliminarly, any significant difference between groups in demographic variables, age, education and gender as well as MMSE score was taken into account. Only education showed a significant differences between groups ($p<0.03$). For avoiding confounding effect, subsequent statistical analyses of variance (ANOVA) were carried out using age, education, gender and MMSE score as covariates. Duncan's test was used for post hoc comparisons. For all statistical test the significance was set to $p<0.05$.

A second session of ANOVA was performed on EEG relative power data. In this analysis, Group factor was the independent variable and frequency band power (delta, theta, alpha1, alpha2, alpha3) the dependent variable.

As successive step, to evaluate the presence of EEG indexes that correlate specifically with vascular damage, we performed statistical analyses to evaluate the specificity of the following ratios: theta/alpha1, using as covariate also TF; alpha2/alpha3 using as covariate also IAF and alpha1/alpha2 with both TF and IAF as covariate. Moreover, we performed correlations (Pearson's moment correlation) between CV damage score and frequency markers (TF and IAF), spectral power, and MMSE. Finally, we performed a control statistical analysis with 4 frequency bands, considering alpha1 and alpha2 as single band (low alpha). This analysis had the aim to verify if the low alpha, when considered as a whole, has the same behavior.

# 3. Results

Figure 1 displays the results for ANOVA analysis of these data showing a significant interaction between Group and Band factors [$F(12.380) = 2.60$); $p < 0.002$] . Interestingly,

Duncan post hoc showed a significant decrease of delta power in G1 compared to G4 ($p < 0.050$) and a significant increase in alpha2 power in G1 compared to G3 and G4 ($p < 0.000$). On the contrary, no differences were found in theta, alpha1 and alpha 3 band power. Moreover, a closer look at the data, in respect to the alpha1 frequency, showed a decrease proportional to the degree of CV damage very similar to alpha2 band, although not significant. On the contrary, in the alpha3 band power this trend was not present, suggesting that vascular damage had no impact on this frequency band.

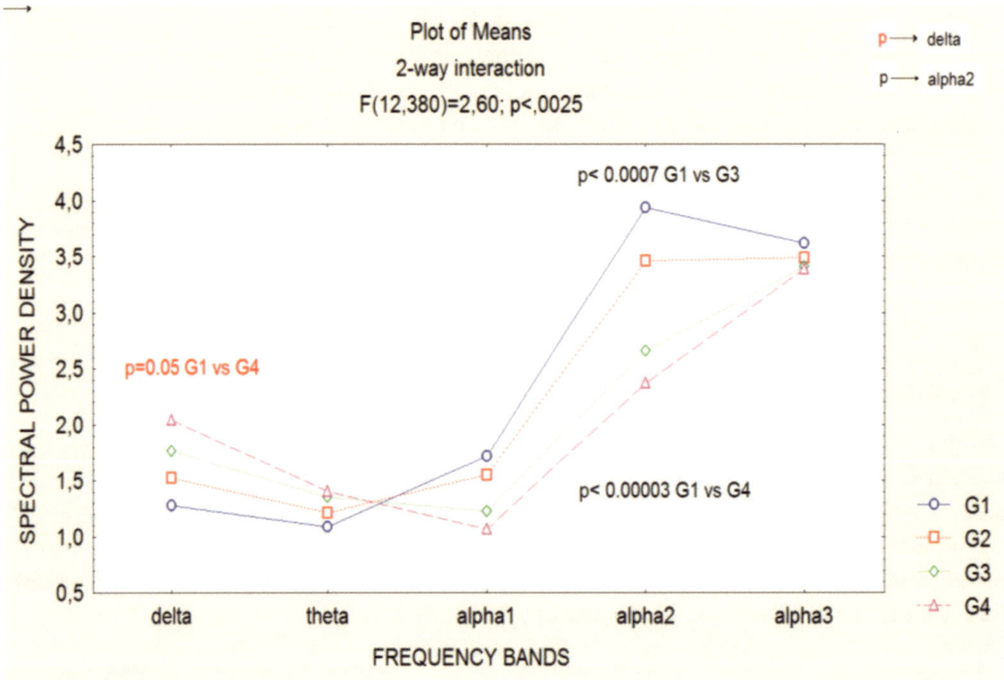


**Figure 1.** Statistical ANOVA interaction among groups, factor and relative band power (delta, theta, alpha1, alpha2, alpha3). In the diagram the difference in delta and alpha2 power among groups is also indicated, based on Duncan's post-hoc testing. (G1, group 1) no vascular damage; (G2, group 2) mild vascular damage; (G3, group 3) moderate vascular damage; (G4, group 4) severe vascular damage (Moretti et al., 2007).

The correlation analysis between CV score and spectral band power showed a significant positive correlation with delta power ($r= 0.221$; $p < 0.03$), a significant negative correlation with alpha1 ($r= -0.312$; $p < 0.002$) and alpha2 power ($r$ -0.363; $p < 0.0003$). The correlations between CV score with theta power ($r= 0.183$; $p = 0.07$) and alpha3 power ($r= -0.002$; $p = 0.93$) were not significant as well as the correlation between CV score and MMSE ($r= -0.07$; $p= 0.4$).

Table 3 displays the values of the theta/alpha1 and alpha2/alpha3 power ratio. The statistical analysis of the theta/alpha1 ratio showed a main effect of Group [$F$ (3.91)=15.51; $p < 0.000$]. Duncan post hoc testing showed a significant increase of the theta/alpha1 ratio between G1 and G2 respect to G3 and G4 ($p < 0.000$). Moreover, the increase of this ratio was significant also between G3 and G4 ($p<0.04$). The statistical analysis of the alpha2/alpha3 power ratio showed a main effect of Group [F (3.91)=4.60; $p < 0.005$]. Duncan post hoc testing showed a significant decrease of the ratio between G1 and G3 ($p < 0.02$), G1 and G4 ($p < 0.010$) and between G2 and G4 ($p < 0.05$). The statistical analysis of the alpha1/alpha2 ratio did not show the main effect of Group ($p < 0.2$).

| | MCI cohort | | Group 1 | Group 2 | Group 3 | p value (ANOVA) |
|---|---|---|---|---|---|---|
| **Number of subjects (f/m)** | 79 (42/37) | | 27 (14/13) | 27 (15/12) | 25 (13/12) | |
| | | | | | | |
| **Age (years)** | 69.2±2.3 | | 66.8±6.8 | 69.4±8.7 | 71.5±6.9 | 0.1 |
| | | | | | | |
| **Education (years)** | 7.7±0.8 | | 8.3±4.5 | 6.7±3.1 | 8.2±4.6 | 0.2 |
| | | | | | | |
| **MMSE** | 27.1±0.4 | | 27.5±1.5 | 27.4±1.5 | 26.6±1.8 | 0.1 |
| | | | | | | |
| **Total AHC volume** | 6965.3±12<br>48.8 | | 8151.2±43<br>6.4 | 7082.7±26<br>6.9 | 5661.8±72<br>0.4 | 0.00001 |
| | | | | | | |
| **AHC-hippocampal volume (mm³)** | 4891.7±90<br>2.6 | | 5771.6±36<br>1.1 | 4935.6±38<br>0.9 | 3967.9±65<br>0.3 | 0.00001 |
| | | | | | | |
| **AHC-amygdalar volume (mm³)** | 2073.5±34<br>8.7 | | 2379.6±32<br>1.3 | 2147.1±30<br>1.3 | 1693.9±28<br>8.5 | 0.0001 |
| | | | | | | |
| **individual hippocampal volume (mm³)** | 4889.8±96<br>2.4 | | 5809.6±31<br>4.2 | 4969.4±25<br>7.6 | 3890.1±55<br>1.4 | 0.00001 |
| | | | | | | |
| **individual amygdalar volume (mm³)** | 2071.7±44<br>6.4 | | 2514.4±25<br>9.5 | 2079.2±12<br>2.8 | 1621.6±18<br>5.2 | 0.0001 |
| | | | | | | |
| **White matter hyperintensities (mm³)** | 3.8±0.5 | | 3.2±2.8 | 4.2±3.8 | 4.1±3.6 | 0.7 |

**Table 3.** Mean values ± standard deviation of sociodemographic characteristics, MMSE scores, white matter hyperintensities, hippocampal and amygdalar volume measurements. Hippocampal and amygdalar volumes are referred to the whole amygdalo-hippocampal complex (AHC) and singularly considered (individual). The t-test refers to AHC vs individual volume in each group.

## 3.1. MRI scans and amygdalo-hippocampal atrophy evaluation

MRI scans were acquired with a 1.0 Tesla Philips Gyroscan at the Neuroradiology Unit of the Città di Brescia hospital, Brescia. The following sequences were used to measure hippocampal and amygdalar volumes: a high-resolution gradient echo T1-weighted sagittal

3D sequence (TR = 20 ms, TE = 5 ms, flip angle = 30°, field of view = 220 mm, acquisition matrix = 256 x 256, slice thickness = 1.3 mm), and a fluid-attenuated inversion recovery (FLAIR) sequence (TR = 5000 ms, TE = 100 ms, flip angle = 90°, field of view = 230 mm, acquisition matrix = 256 x 256, slice thickness = 5 mm). Hippocampal, amygdalar and white matter hyperintensities (WMHs) volumes were obtained for each subject. The hippocampal and amygdalar boundaries were manually traced on each hemisphere by a single tracer with the software program DISPLAY (McGill University, Montreal, Canada) on contiguous 1.5 mm slices in the coronal plane. The amygdala is an olive-shaped mass of gray matter located in the superomedial part of the temporal lobe, partly superior and anterior to the hippocampus. The starting point for amygdala tracing was at the level where it is separated from the entorhinal cortex by intrarhinal sulcus, or tentorial indentation, which forms a marked indent at the site of the inferior border of the amygdala. The uncinate fasciculus, at the level of basolateral nuclei groups, was considered as the anterior-lateral border. The amygdalo-striatal transition area, which is located between lateral amygdaloid nucleus and ventral putamen, was considered as the posterior-lateral border. The posterior end of amygdaloid nucleus was defined as the point where gray matter starts to appear superior to the alveolus and laterally to the hippocampus. If the alveolus was not visible, the inferior horn of the lateral ventricle was employed as border (Moretti et al., 2008). The starting point for hippocampus tracing was defined as the hippocampal head when it first appears below the amygdala, the alveus defining the superior and anterior border of the hippocampus. The fimbria was included in the hippocampal body, while the grey matter rostral to the fimbria was excluded. The hippocampal tail was traced until it was visible as an oval shape located caudally and medially to the trigone of the lateral ventricles (Moretti et al., 2007a,b). The intraclass correlation coefficients were 0.95 for the hippocampus and 0.83 for the amygdala.

White matter hyperintensities (WMHs) were automatically segmented on the FLAIR sequences by using previously described algorithms (Moretti et al., 2007a,b). Briefly, the procedure includes (i) filtering of FLAIR images to exclude radiofrequency inhomogeneities, (ii) segmentation of brain tissue from cerebrospinal fluid, (iii) modelling of brain intensity histogram as a gaussian distribution and (iv) classification of the voxels whose intensities were ≥3.5 SDs above the mean as WMHs (Moretti et al., 2007a,b) Total WMHs volume was computed by counting the number of voxels segmented as WMHs and multiplying by the voxel size (5 $mm^3$). To correct for individual differences in head size, hippocampal, amygdalar and WMHs volumes were normalized to the total intracranial volume (TIV), obtained by manually tracing with DISPLAY the entire intracranial cavity on 7 mm thick coronal slices of the T1 weighted images. Both manual and automated methods user here have advantages and disadvantages. Manual segmentation of the hippocampus and amygdala is currently considered the gold standard technique for the measurement of such complex structures. The main disadvantages of manual tracing are that it is operator dependent and time consuming. Conversely, automated techniques are more reliable and less time-consuming, but may be less accurate when dealing with structures without clearly identifiable borders. This however is not the case for WMHs which appear as hyperintense on FLAIR sequences.

Left and right hippocampal as well as amygdalar volumes were estimated and summed to obtain a total volume (individual) of both anatomical structures. In turn, total amygdalar and hippocampal volume were summed obtaining the whole AHC volume. AHC (whole) volume has been divided in tertiles obtaining three groups. In each group hippocampal and amygdalar volume (within AHC) has been computed. The last volumes were compared with the previous obtained individual (hippocampal and amygdalar) volumes.

### 3.2. Statistical analysis and data management

The analysis of variance (ANOVA) has been applied as statistical tool. At first, any significant differences among groups in demographic variables, i.e., age, education, MMSE score, and morphostructural characteristics, i.e., AHC, hippocampal, amygdalar and white matter hyperintensities (WMHs) volume were evaluated (table 1). Greenhouse-Geisser correction and Mauchley's sphericity test were applied to all ANOVAs. In order to avoid a confounding effect, ANOVAs were carried out using age, education, MMSE score, and WMHs as covariates. Duncan's test was used for post-hoc comparisons. For all statistical tests the significance level was set at $p<0.05$.

At first, we choose to focus the changes of brain rhythmicity induced from hippocampal atrophy alone. ,Subjects were subdivided in four groups based on hippocampal volume of a normal, control sample matched for age, sex and education as compared to the whole MCI group. In the normal group the ratio female/male was 93/46, mean age was 68.9 (SD ±10.3) mean education years 8.9 (SD ±9.4). The mean and standard deviation of the hippocampal volume in the normal old population of 139 subjects were 5.72 ± 1.1 cm3 . In this way, 4 groups were obtained: the no atrophy group with hippocampal volume equal or superior to the normal mean (total hippocampal volume from 6.79 cm3 to 5.75 cm3; G1); the mild atrophy group which has hippocampal volume within 1.5 SD below the mean of hippocampal normal control value (total hippocampal volume from 5.70 to 4.70 cm3; G2); the moderate atrophy group which has hippocampal volume between 1.5 and 3 SD below the mean of normal hippocampus (total hippocampal volume from 4.65 to 3.5 cm3; G3); and the severe atrophy group which has hippocampal volume between 3 and 4.5 SD below the mean of hippocampal normal control volume (total hippocampal volume from 3.4 to 2.53 cm3; G4). The rationale for the selection of 1,5 SD was to obtain reasonably pathological groups based on hippocampal volume. A SD below 1.5 could recollect still normal population based on hippocampal volume. On the other side, a SD over 1.5 could not allow an adequate size of all subgroups in study.

Subsequently, ANOVA was performed in order to verify 1) the difference of AHC volume among groups; 2) the difference of hippocampal and amygdalar volume within AHC among groups; 3) the difference of hippocampal and amygdalar volume individually considered among groups; 4) NPS impairment based on ACH atrophy.

Moreover, as a control analysis, in order to detect if difference in EEG markers was linked to significant difference in volume measurements, the volume of hippocampus within AHC was compared with the hippocampal volume individually considered, as well as the amygdalar volume within AHC was compared with the amygdalar volume individually considered. This control analysis was performed through a paired t-test.

Subsequently, ANOVA was performed in order to check differences in theta/gamma and alpha3/alpha2 relative power ratio in the three groups ordered by decreasing tertile values of the whole AHC volume. In each ANOVA, group was the independent variable, the frequency ratios was the dependent variable and age, education, MMSE score, and WMHs was used as covariates. Duncan's test was used for post-hoc comparisons. For all statistical tests the significance level was set at $p<0.05$.

In order to check closer association with EEG markers, hippocampal volume, and amygdalar volume within AHC were analyzed separately. A control analysis was carried out also on the individual hippocampal and amygdalar volumes based on decreasing tertile values for homogeneity with the main analysis.

## 4. Results

Figure 2 displays the results for ANOVA analysis performed on 4 groups of MCI considering growing values of hippocampal atrphy. The results show a significant interaction between Group and Band power [$F(12,336)= 2,36$); $p < 0.007$]. Duncan post hoc showed that G3 group has the highest alpha2 and alpha3 power statistically significant with respect to all other groups ($p<0.05$; $p< 0.006$ respectively). The same trend was present in the subsidiary ANOVA. These results show that the relationship between hippocampal atrophy and EEG relative power is not proportional to the hippocampal atrophy and highlight that the group with a moderate hippocampal volume had a particular pattern of EEG activity as compared to all other groups.

Table 2 summarizes the ANOVA results of demographic variables, i.e., age, education, MMSE score, and morphostructural characteristics, i.e., hippocampal, amygdalar and white matter hyperintensities volume in the whole MCI cohort as well as in the three subgroups in study. Hippocampal and aymgdalar volumes are considered as parts of the whole AHC volume as well as individually considered. Significant statistical results were found in hippocampal and amygdalar volume both within the AHC (respectively, $F_{2,76}$=92.74; $p<0.00001$ and $F_{2,76}$=33.82; $p<0.00001$) and individually considered (respectively, $F_{2,76}$=157.27; $p<0.00001$ and $F_{2,76}$=132.5; $p<0.00001$). The global AHC volume also showed significant results ($F_{2,76}$=159.27; $p<0.00001$). Duncan's post-hoc test showed a significant increase ($p< 0.01$) in all comparisons. The paired t-test showed significant difference between the volume of ACH-amygdala vs amygdalar volume individually considered in the first group ($p <0.03$). The amygdalar volume difference in the other groups (respectively $p=0.2$ and 0.1) as well as the difference in the volume of AHC-hippocampus vs individual hippocampus ($p= 0.4$ in the first, $p=0.5$ in the second and $p=0.1$ in the third group) was not statistically significant.

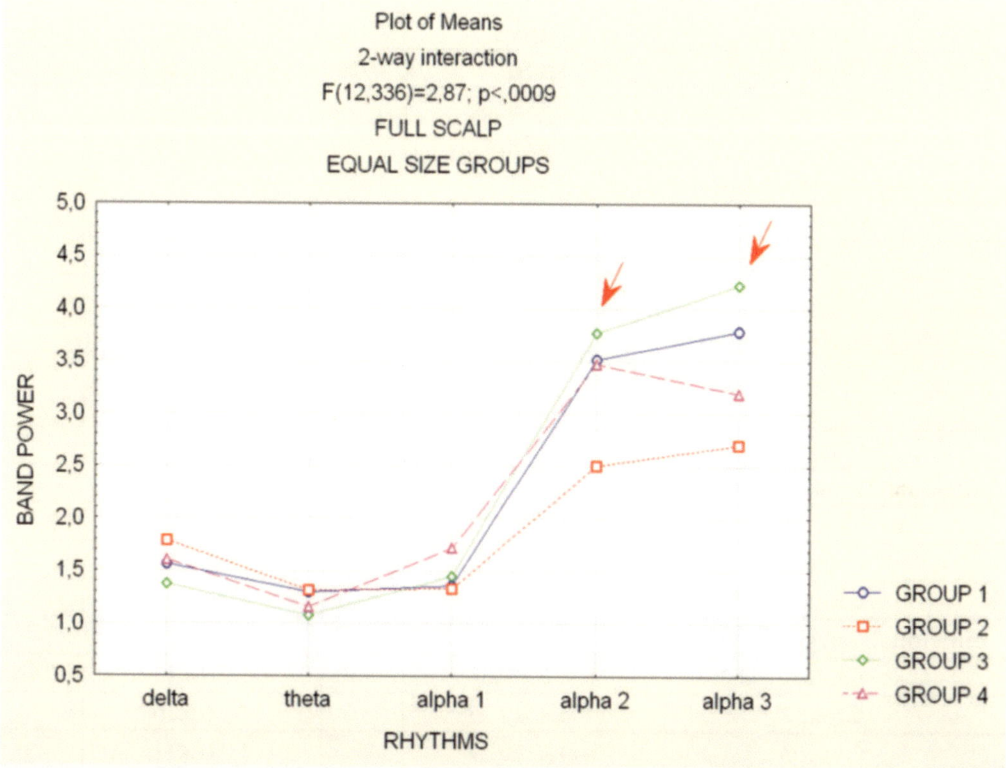


**Figure 2.** Statistical ANOVA interaction among Group factors, and relative band powers (delta, theta, alpha1, alpha2, alpha3), on the full scalp region. The groups are based on mean and standard deviations in a normal elderly sample. Group 1, no hippocampal atrophy; Group 2, mild hippocampal atrophy; Group 3, moderate hippocampal atrophy; Group 4 severe hippocampal atrophy. Post-hoc results are indicated in the diagram (see Moretti et al., 2007).

Table 3 and 4 shows the results of theta/gamma and alpha3/alpha2 ratio in the groups based on the decrease of whole AHC volume as well as, within the same group, the decrease of hippocampal and amygdalar volumes separately considered. ANOVA shows results towards significance when amygdalo-ippocampal volume is considered globally both in theta/gamma ($F_{2,76}$ =2.77; $p<0.06$) and alpha3/alpha2 ratio ($F_{2,76}$ =2.71; $p<0.07$). When amygdalar and hippocampal volumes were considered separately, ANOVA results revealed significant main effect Group, respectively, in theta/gamma ratio analysis ($F_{2,76}$ =3.46; $p<0.03$) for amygdalar and alpha3/alpha2 ratio for hippocampal ($F_{2,76}$=3.38; $p<0.03$) decreasing volume. The ANOVA did not show significant results in theta/gamma ratio when considering hippocampal volume ($F_{2,76}$=0.3; $p<0.7$) and in alpha3/alpha2 ratio when considering amygdalar volume ($F_{2,76}$=1.46; $p<0.2$). The control analysis (individual volumes) did not show any significant result neither for hippocampal (theta/gamma, $F_{2,76}$=0.3; $p<0.7$; alpha3/alpha2, $F_{2,76}$=2.15; $p<0.1$) nor for amygdalar volume (theta/gamma, $F_{2,76}$=0.76; $p<0.4$; alpha3/alpha2, $F_{2,76}$=2.15; $p<0.1$).

| Hippocampal + amygdalar volume | theta/gamma ratio ($\mu v^2$) | p value | alpha3/alpha2 ratio ($\mu v^2$) | p value |
|---|---|---|---|---|
| Group1 | 1.40±0.35 | 0.06 | 1.05±0.11 | 0.07 |
| Group2 | 1.43±0.35 | | 1.11±0.14 | |
| Group3 | 1.47±0.44 | | 1.12±0.16 | |
| **AHC-hippocampal volume** | | | | |
| Group1 | 1.39±0.27 | 0.7 | 1.04±0.11 | 0.03 |
| Group2 | 1.48±0.45 | | 1.11±0.15 | |
| Group3 | 1.43±0.41 | | 1.12±0.14 | |
| **AHC-amygdalar volume** | | | | |
| Group1 | 1.36±0.37 | 0.03 | 1.04±0.13 | 0.2 |
| Group2 | 1.44±0.36 | | 1.12±0.16 | |
| Group3 | 1.49±0.39 | | 1.09±0.11 | |
| **individual hippocampal volume** | | | | |
| Group1 | 1.39±0.27 | 0.7 | 1.04±0.11 | 0.1 |
| Group2 | 1.48±0.45 | | 1.07±0.15 | |
| Group3 | 1.43±0.40 | | 1.10±0.14 | |
| **individual amygdalar volume** | | | | |
| Group1 | 1.39±0.37 | 0.1 | 1.04±0.13 | 0.4 |
| Group2 | 1.43±0.36 | | 1.12±0.16 | |
| Group3 | 1.46±0.39 | | 1.09±0.11 | |

**Table 4.** Relative power band ratios in amygdalo-hippocampal complex (AHC), hippocampal and amygdalar atrophy. Hippocampal and amygdalar volumes are referred to the whole amygdalo-hippocampal complex (AHC) and singularly considered (individual).

## 4.1. Clinical and neurophsyiological remarks

### *4.1.1. MCI and EEG markers: degenerative versus vascular impairment*

A large body of literature has previously demonstrated that in subjects with cognitive decline is present an increase of theta relative power (Moretti et al 2007a,b, 2008), a decrease of gamma relative power (Stam et al., 2003, Moretti et al., 2007a,b 2008) as well as an increase of high alpha as compared to low alpha band (Moretti et al., 2008). On the whole theta/gamma ratio and alpha3/alpha2 ratio could be considered reliable EEG markers of cognitive decline.

The amygdalo-hippocampal network is a key structure in the generation of theta rhythm. More specifically, theta synchronization is increased between LA and CA1 region of hippocampus during long-term memory retrieval, but not during short-term or remote memory retrieval (Seidenbecher et al., 2003; Narayanan et al., 2007). In particular, the AHC is critically involved in the formation and retention of fear memories (Narayanan et al., 2007). Theta synchronization in AHC appears to be a neural correlate of fear, apt to improve the neural communication during memory retrieval (Narayanan et al., 2007). On the other hand, the retrieval of hippocampus-dipendent memory is provided by the integrity of CA3-CA1 interplay coordinated by gamma oscillations (Montgomery and Buzsaki, 2007). Our results confirm and extends all previous findings. The atrophy of AHC determines increasing memory deficits. The brain oscillatory activity of this MCI state is characterized by an increase of theta/gamma ratio and alpha3/alpha2 relative power ratio, confirming the overall reliability of these EEG markers in cognitive decline. Our results suggest that theta synchronization is mainly due to the amygdala activation or as a subsequent final net effect within the AHC functioning driven by the amygdala excitation. The increase in theta activities in AHC, representing an increase in neuronal communication apt to promote or stabilize synaptic plasticity in relation to the effort to retention of associative memories (Sauseng et al., 2004), could be active also during an ongoing degenerative process. The excitation mechanism could be facilitated by the loss of GABA inhibitory process, determining the decrease of gamma rhythm generation (Bragin et al., 1995; Montgomery and Buzsaki, 2007).

As regards the CV damage, our results showed that the CV damage affected both delta and low alpha band power (alpha1 and alpha2). In the delta band we observed a power increase proportional to the CV damage, with a significant increase in the group with severe CV damage, as compared to the no-CV-damage group. The impact of the CV damage on the delta power was confirmed by the significant positive correlation between CV damage score and delta power itself.

The increase in the delta band power could be explained as a progressive cortical disconnection due to the slowing of the conduction along cortico-subcortical connecting pathways.

This result confirmed the increase in the delta band power we had observed in CV patients, as compared to normal elderly subjects (Moretti et al., 2004). It is to be noted that the increase in the delta band power reflects a global state of cortical deafferentation, due to various anatomofunctional substrates, such as stages of sleep, metabolic encephalopathy or cortico-thalamocortical dysrhythmia (Llinas et al., 1999). In the low a band power, we observed a significant decrease in the a2 band power for the groups with moderate and severe CV damage, as compared to the no-CV-damage group. In the a1 frequency band, there was a similar decrease although it did not reach statistically significant values. These results were confirmed by a correlation analysis which showed a significant negative correlation between CV damage score and a1 and a2 band powers. In our results, the CV damage did not show any impact on the a3 (or high a) power. This is a confirmation of what we found in the previous study, where no differences between VaD patients and normal elderly (but not in AD vs normal elderly) subjects were detected in the a3 power.

Together, these results could suggest different generators for low a and high a frequency bands. In particular, the low a band power could affect cortico-subcortical mechanisms, such as cortico-thalamic, cortico-striatal and cortico-basal ones. This could explain the sensitivity of the low a frequency band to subcortical vascular damage. On the contrary, the a3 band power could affect to a greater extent those cortico-cortical interactions based on synaptic efficiency prone to degenerative rather than CV damages (Klimesch, 1999; Klimesch et al., 2007). In order to find reliable indices of CV damage, we checked the theta/a1 band power ratio. Previous studies have shown the reliability of this kind of approach in quantitative EEG in demented patients (Jelic et al., 1997). The importance of this ratio lies in the presence of such frequency bands on the opposite side of the TF, that is, the EEG frequency index most significantly affected by the CV damage. So, the theta/a1 band power ratio could represent the most sensitive EEG marker of CV damage. The results showed a significant increase of the theta/a1 band power ratio in moderate and severe CV damage groups, as compared to mild and no-CV-damage groups. This ratio increase establishes a proportional increase of the theta band power relative to the a1 band power with respect to the CV damage, even though a significant increase in the h band power per se (or a decrease in the a1 band power per se) is not present. This could suggest a reliable specificity for the theta/a1 band power ratio in focusing the presence of a subcortical CV damage.

#### *4.1.2. MCI , cognitive deficits (memory and attention) and EEG activity*

The vulnerability and damage of the connections of hippocampus with amygdala could affect reconsolidation of long-term memory and give rise to memory deficits and behavioural symptoms. Several experiments shows that amygdala activity is prominent during period of intense arousal, e.g. the anticipation of a noxious stimulus (Parè et al., 2002) or the maintenance of vigilance to negative stimuli (Garolera et al., 2007). So far, the theta synchronization induced by the amygdala is deeply involved in endogenous attentional mechanism. Interestingly, the increase of high alpha synchronization has been found in internally-cued mechanisms of attention, associated with inhibitory top-down processes (Klimesch, 2007). Of note, the amygdala is intimately involved in the anatomo-physiological anterior pathways of attention through its connections with anterior cingulated cortex, anteroventral, anteromedial and pulvinar thalamic nuclei (Young et al., 2007). The particular role of amygdala in negative human emotions could indicate that AHC atrophy is associated with excessive level of subcortical inputs not adequately filtered by attentive processing, determining fear and anxiety and generating cognitive interference in memory performance. Of note, an altered emotional response is very frequent in MCI patients (Ellison et al., 2008, Rozzini et al., 2008). In a feed-back process, this alteration could determine a general state of "hyperattention" during which top-down internal processes prevail on the bottom-up phase, altering attention mechanism and preventing a correct processing of sensory stimuli. Focused attention has been found impaired in MCI patients in particular when they have to benefit from a cue stimulus (Johanssen et al., 1999; Berardi et al., 2005 ; Levinoff et al., 2005 Tales et al. 2005a, 2005b). This particular state could be useful for maintain a relatively spared global cognitive performance, whereas it could fail when a detailed analysis of a sensory stimulus is required. This "hyperattentive" state could represent the attempt to recollect memory and/or spatial traces from hippocampus and to combine them within associative areas connected with hippocampus itself.

The increase of alpha3/alpha2 ratio in our results support the concomitance of anterior attentive mechanism impairment in subject with MCI, even though there are not overt clinical deficits. The mayor association of the increase of alpha3/alpha2 ratio with the hippocampal formation within the AHC, suggest that this filter activity is carried out by hippocampus and its input-output connections along anterior attentive circuit and AHC. Interestingly, a recent work has demonstrated that the mossy fiber (MF) pathway of the hippocampus connects the dentate gyrus to the auto-associative CA3 network, and the information it carries is controlled by a feedforward circuit combining disynaptic inhibition with monosynaptic excitation. Analysis of the MF associated circuit revealed that this circuit could act as a highpass filter (Zalay and Bardakjian, 2006).

The natural history of a group of subjects at very high-risk for developing dementia due to subcortical vascular damage [subcortical vascular MCI (svMCI)] has recently been described (Frisoni et al., 2002; Galluzzi et al., 2005). In such study, MCI patients with CV etiology developed a distinctive clinical phenotype characterized by poor performance on frontal tests, and neurological features of parkinsonism without tremor (impairment of balance and gait).These clinical features could be explained by our results. In CV patients, we observed a slowing of the a frequency in the two groups with greater CV damage, as compared to the groups with lesser CV damage. This is in line with a previous study (Moretti et al., 2004) showing that the major effect of the CV damage, in patients with vascular dementia (VaD) vs normal elderly and Alzheimer's patients. A reasonable (although speculative) explanation of the present results is that the CV damage-induced slowing of the a frequency start point could be mainly attributed to the lowering of the conduction time of synaptic action potentials throughout cortico-subcortical fibers, such as cortico-basal or cortico-thalamic pathways (Steriade and Llinas, 1988). In fact, experimental models have previously shown that the EEG frequency is due to axonal delay and synaptic time of cortico-subcortical interactions (Lopes da Silva et al., 1976; Nunez et al., 2001; Doiron et al., 2003). Most interestingly, other studies have demonstrated that fiber myelination affects the speed propagation along cortical fibers, and that this parameter is strictly correlated to the frequency range recorded on the scalp. In fact, a theoretical model considering a mean speed propagation in white matter fibers of 7.5 m/s (together with other parameters) is associated with a fundamental mode frequency of 9 Hz (Nunez and Srinivasan, 2006), that is, the typical mode of scalp-recorded EEG. It is to be noted that a correlation between white matter damage and widespread slowing of EEG rhythmicity was found in other studies, following the presence of cognitive decline (Szelies et al., 1999), multiple sclerosis (Leocani et al., 2000), or cerebral tumors (Goldensohn, 1979). In order to find reliable indices of CV damage, we checked the theta/a1 band power ratio. Previous studies have shown the reliability of this kind of approach in quantitative EEG in demented patients (Jelic et al., 1997). The importance of this ratio lies in the presence of such frequency bands on the opposite side of the TF, that is, the EEG frequency index most significantly affected by the CV damage. So, the theta/a1 band power ratio could represent the most sensitive EEG marker of CV damage. The results showed a significant increase of the theta/a1 band power ratio in moderate and severe CV damage groups, as compared to mild and no-CV-damage groups. This ratio increase establishes a proportional increase of the theta band power relative to the a1 band power with respect to the CV damage, even though a significant increase in the theta band power per se (or a decrease in the a1 band power per se) is not present. This could suggest a reliable specificity for the theta/alpha1 band power ratio in focusing the presence of a subcortical CV damage.

## Author details

D. V. Moretti*, G. B. Frisoni, G. Binetti and O. Zanetti
*IRCCS S. Giovanni di Dio Fatebenefratelli, Brescia; Italy*

## 5. References

Albert M, Smith LA, Scherr PA, Taylor JO, Evans DA, Funkenstein HH (1991) Use of brief cognitive tests to identify individuals in the community with clinically diagnosed Alzheimer's disease. *Int J Neurosci* 57, (3–4):167–78.

Amodio P, Wenin H, Del Piccolo F, Mapelli D, Montagnese S, Pellegrini A, Musto C, Gatta A, Umiltà C (2002) Variability of trail making test, symbol digit test and line trait test in normal people. A normative study taking into account age-dependent decline and sociobiological variables. *Aging Clin Exp Res* 14, 117–131.

Arnold SE, Hyman BT, Flory J, Damasco AR, Van Hoesen GW. The topographical and neuroanatomical distribution od neurofibrillaty tangles and neuritic plaques in the cerebral cortex of patients with Alzheimer's disease. Cereb Cortex 1991; 1: 103-116.

Babiloni C, Binetti G, Cassetta E, Dal Forno G, Del Percio C, Ferreri F, Ferri R, Frisoni G, Hirata K, Lanuzza B, Miniussi C, Moretti DV, Nobili F, Rodriguez G, Romani GL, Salinari S, Rossini PM. Sources of cortical rhythms change as a function of cognitive impairment in pathological aging: a multi-centric study. Clin Neurophysiol 2006 a;117(2):252–68.

Basso A, Capitani E, Laiacona M (1987) Raven's coloured progressive matrices: normative values on 305 adult normal controls. *Funct Neurol* 2, 189–194.

Bennett DA, Schneider JA, Bienais JL, Evans DA, Wilson RS. Mild cognitive impairment is related to Alzheimer disease pathology and cerebral infarctions. Neurology, 2004; 23:325-335.

Berardi AM, Parasuraman R, Haxby JV. Sustained attentino in mild Alzheimer's disease. Dev Neuropsychol 2005; 58: 507-537.

Bobinski M, Wegiel J, Wisniewski HM, Tarnawski M, Reisberg B, Mlozidc B *et al.*, Atrophy of hippocampal formation subdivisions correlates with stage and duration of Alzheimer's disease. Dementia 1995; 6: 205-210.

Bragin A, Jando G, Nadasdy Z, Hetke J, Wise K, Buzsaki G. Gamma (40-100 Hz) oscillation in the hippocampus of the behaving rat. Journal of neuroscience 1995; 15: 47-60.

Caffarra P, Vezzadini G, Dieci F, Zonato F, Venneri A (2002) Rey- Osterrieth complex figure: normative values in an Italian population sample. *Neurol Sci* 22, 443–437.

* Corresponding Author

Callen Dj, Black SE, Gao F, Caldwell CB, Szalai JP. Beyond the hippocampus: MRI volumetry confirms widespread limbic atrophy in AD. Neurology 2001; 57: 1669-1674.

Carlesimo GA, Caltagirone C, Gainotti G (1996) The Mental Deterioration Battery: normative data, diagnostic reliability and qualitative analyses of cognitive impairment. The Group for the Standardization of the Mental Deterioration Battery. *Eur Neurol* 36, 378–384.

De Curtis M, Parè D. The rhinal cortices : a wall of inhibitio between the neocortex and the hippocampus. Progress in neurobiology 2004; 74: 101-110.

Della Maggiore V, Chau W, Peres-Neto PR, Mclntosh AR. An empirical comparison of SPM preprocessing parameters to the analysis of fMRI data. Neuroimage 2002; 17; 19-28.

Dickerson BC, Salat DH, Bates JF, Atiya M, Kiliiany RJ, Greve DN *et al.* Medial temporal lobe function and structure in midl cognitive impairment. Ann Neurol 2004; 56: 27-35.

Dickerson BC, Salat DH, Greve DN, Chua EF Rand-Giovannetti E, Rentz DM *et al.*Increased hippomcapal activation in midl cognitive impairment compared to normal aging and AD. Neurology 2005; 65: 404-411.

Doiron B, Chacron MJ, Maler L, Longtin L, Bastian J. Inhibitory feedback required for network oscillatory responses to communication but not prey stimuli. Nature 2003;421:538–43.

Du AT, Schuff N, Amend D, Laasko MP, Hsu YY, Jagust WJ *et al.* magnetic resonance imaging of the enthorinal cortex and hippocampus in mild cognitive impairment and Alzheimer's disease. J Neurol Neurosurg Psychiatry 2001; 71: 441-7.

Ellison JM, Harper DG, Berlow Y, Zeranski L. Beyond the "C" in MCI: noncognitive symptoms in amnestic and non-amnestic mild cognitive impairment. CNS Spectr. 2008 Jan;13(1):66-72.

Ferreri F, Pauri F, Pasqualetti P, Fini R, Dal Forno G, Rossini PM. Motor cortex excitability in Alzheimer's disease: a transcranial magnetic stimulation study. Ann Neurol. 2003 Jan;53(1):102-8.

Flicker CS, Ferris H, Reisberg B. Mild cognitive impairment in the elderly: predictors of dementia. Neurology 1991;41:1006–9.etersen RC, Smith GE, Ivnik RJ, Tangalos EG, Schaid SN, Thibodeau SN, Kokmen E, Waring SC, Kurland LT. Apolipoprotein E status as a predictor of the development of Alzheimer's disease in memoryimpaired individuals. J Am Med Assoc 1995;273:1274–8.

Folstein MF, Folstein SE, McHugh PR (1975) 'Mini mental state': a practical method for grading the cognitive state of patients for clinician. *J Psychiatr Res* 12, 189–98.

Frisoni GB, Galluzzi S, Bresciani L, Zanetti O, Geroldi C. Mild cognitive impairment with subcortical vascular features: Clinical characteristics and outcome. J Neurol 2002; 249: 1423–1432.

Frisoni GB, Galluzzi S, Bresciani L, Zanetti O, Geroldi C. Mild cognitive impairment with subcortical vascular features: Clinical characteristics and outcome. J Neurol 2002; 249: 1423–1432.

Frisoni GB, Prestia A, Rasser PE, Bonetti M, Thompson PM. In vivo mapping of incremental cortical atrophy from incipient to overt Alzheimer's disease. *J Neurol.* 2009 Feb 28. [Epub ahead of print]

Galluzzi S, Sheu CF, Zanetti O, Frisoni G B. Distinctive Clinical Features of Mild Cognitive Impairment with Subcortical CV Disease. Dement Geriatr Cogn Disord 2005;19:196–203

Garolera M, Coppola R, Muñoz KE, Elvevåg B, Carver FW, Weinberger DR, Goldberg TE. Amygdala activation in affective priming: a magnetoencephalogram study. Neuroreport. 2007 Sep 17;18(14):1449-53.

Geroldi C, Rossi R, Calvagna C, Testa C, Bresciani L, Binetti G, Zanetti O, Frisoni GB (2006) Medial temporal atrophy but not memory deficit predicts progression to dementia in patients with mild cognitive impairment. *J Neurol. Neurosurg. Psychiatry* 77, 1219-1222.

Gloveli T, Dugladze T, Rotstein HG, Traub RD, Monyer H, Heinemann U, Whittington MA, Kopell NJ. Orthogonal arrangement of rhythm-generating microcircuits in the hippocampus. 2005; 13295-13300.

Gold G, Bouras C, Kovari E, Canito A, Glaria BG, Malky A, *et al.* Clinical validità of Braak neuropathological staging in the oldest-old. Acta neuropathol 2000, 99: 579-582.

Goldensohn ES. Use of EEG for evaluation of focal intracranial lesions. In: Klass DW, Daly DD, editors. Current practice of clinical electroencephalography. New York: Raven; 1979. p. 307–41.

Golob EJ, Irimajiri R. Starr A. Auditory cortical activity in amnestic mild cognitive impairment: relationship to subtype and conversion to dementia. Brain 2007; 130:740-752.

Hamalainen A, Pihlaimaki M, Tanila H, Hanninen T, Niskanen E, Tervo S, Karjalainen PA, Vanninen RL, Soininen H. Increased fMRI responses during encoding in mild cognitive impairment, Neurobiology of Aging (2006), doi:10.1016/j.neurobiolaging.2006.08.008

Huang C, Wahlund LO, Dierks T, Julin P, Winblad B, Jelic V. Discrimination of Alzheimer's disease and mild cognitive impairment by equivalent EEG sources: a cross-sectional and longitudinal study. Clin Neurophysiol 2000;11:1961–7.

Hughes CP, Berg L, Danziger WL, Cohen LA, Martin RL (1982) A new clinical rating scale for the staging of dementia. *BrJ Psychiatry* 140, 1225–30.

Jelic V, Johansson SE, Almkvist O, Shigeta M, Julin P, Nordberg A, Winblad B, Wahlund LO. Quantitative electroencephalography in mild cognitive impairment: longitudinal changes and possible prediction of Alzheimer's disease. Neurobiol Aging 2000;21(4):533–40.

Jelic V, Julin P, Shigeta M, Nordberg A, Lannfelt L, Winblad B, Wahlund LO. Apolipoprotein E ε4 allele decreases functional connectivity in Alzheimer's disease as measured by EEG coherence. Journal of Neurology, Neurosurgery, and Psychiatry 1997;63:59–65.

Jiang Z. Study on EEG power and coherence in patients with mild cognitive impairment during working memory task. Journal of Zhejiang University SCIENCE B 2005; 6: 1213-1219.

Jiang Z., Zheng L. Inter and intra-hemispheric EEG coherence in patients with mild cognitive impairment at rest and during working memory task. Journal of Zhejiang University SCIENCE B 2006; 5: 357-364.

Johannsen P, Jacobsen J, Bruhn P, Gjedde A. Cortical responses to sustained and divided attention in Alzheimer's disease. Neuroimage 1999; 10: 269-281.

Johnson JD. The conversational brain: fronto-hippocampal interaction and disconnection. Medical Hypotheses 2006; 67: 759-764.

Klimesch W, Sauseng P, Hanslmayr S. EEG alpha oscillations: The inhibition timing hypothesis. Brain Res Rev 2007; 53: 63-88.

Klimesch W. EEG alpha and theta oscillations reflect cognitive and memory performance: a review and analysis. Brain Res Rev 1999;29: 169–95.

Koenig T, Prichep L, Dierks T, Hubl D, Wahlund LO, John ER, Jelic V. Decreased EEG synchronization in Alzheimer's disease and mild cognitive impairment. Neurobiol Aging 2005;26(2):165–71.

Kramer JH, Reed BR, Mungas D, Weiner MW, Chui HC. Executive dysfunction in subcortical ischaemic vascular disease. J Neurol Neurosurg Psychiatry 2002;72:217– 20.

Lavenex P, Amaral DG. Hippocampal-neocortical interaction: a hierarchy of associativity. Hippocampus 2000; 10:420-430.

Lawton MP, Brodie EM (1969) Assessment of older people: self maintaining and instrumental activity of daily living. *J Gerontol*. 9,179–86.

Leocani L, Locatelli T, Martinelli V, Rovaris M, Falautano M, Filippi M, Magnani G, Comi G. Electroencephalographic coherence analysis in multiple sclerosis: correlation with clinical, neuropsychological, and MRI findings. J Neurol Neurosurg Psychiatry 2000; 69:192–8.

Levinoff EJ, Saumier D, Chertkow H. Focused attention deficits in patients with Alzheimer's disease and midl cognitive impairment. Brain and cognition 2005; 57: 127-130.

Llinas RR, Ribary U, Jeanmonod D, Kronberg E, Mitra PP. Thalamocortical dysrhythmia: a neurological and neuropsychiatric syndrome characterized by magnetoencephalography. Proc Natl Acad Sci USA 1999;96(26):15222–7.

Lopes da Silva FH, van Rotterdam A, Barts P, van Heusden E, Burr W. Models of neuronal populations: the basic mechanism of rhythmicity. In: Corner MA, Swaab DF, editors. Perspectives of brain research. Progress in brain research, vol. 45. Amsterdam: Elsevier; 1976. p. 281–308.

Machulda MM, Ward HA, Borowski B, Gunter JL, Cha RH, O'Brien Pc, *et al.*, Comparison od memory fMRI response among normal, MCI, and Alzheimer's patients. Neurology 2003; 61: 500-506.

Montgomery SM, Buzsaki G. Gamma oscillations dynamically couple hippocampal CA3 and CA1 regions during memory task performance. PNAS, 2007; 104: 14495-14500.

Moretti D.V., Fracassi C., Pievani M., Geroldi C., Binetti G., Zanetti O., Sosta K., Rossini P. M. Frisoni G. B., 2009. Increase of theta/gamma ratio is associated with memory impairment. Clin. Neurophysiol. 120(2), 295-303

Moretti D.V., Pievani M., Fracassi C., Binetti G., Rosini S., Geroldi C., Zanetti O., Rossini P.M., Frisoni G.B., 2008. Increase of theta/gamma and alpha3/alpha2 ratio is associated with amygdalo-hippocampal complex atrophy. J. Alzheimer Disease, 120 (2), 295-303.

Moretti DV, Babiloni C, Binetti G, Cassetta E, Dal Forno G, Ferreri F, Ferri R, Lanuzza B, Miniussi C, Nobili F, Rodriguez G, Salinari S, Rossini PM. Individual analysis of EEG frequency and band power in mild Alzheimer's disease. Clin Neurophysiol 2004;115:299–308.

Moretti DV, Miniussi C, Frisoni GB, Geroldi C, Zanetti O, Binetti G, Rossini PM (2007a) Hippocampal atrophy and EEG markers in subjects with mild cognitive impairment. *Clinical neurophysiology* 118, 2716-2729.

Moretti DV, Miniussi C, Frisoni GB, Zanetti O, Binetti G, Geroldi C, Galluzzi S, Rossini PM (2007b) Vascular damage and EEG markers in subjects with mild cognitive impairment. *Clinical Neurophysiolog.* 118, 1866-1876.

Narayanan RT, Seidenbecher T, Sangha S, Stork O, Pape HC. Theta resynchronization during reconsolidation of remote contextual fear memory. Neuroreport. 2007 Jul 16;18(11):1107-11.

Nestor PJ, Scheltens P, Hodges JR. Advances in early detection of Alzheimer's disease. *Nature Medicine* 2004; 10: 34–41

Nunez PL, Srinivasan R. A theoretical basis for standing and traveling brain waves, Clinical Neurophysiology 2006; 117 (11): 2425-2435Szelies B, Mielke R, Kessler J, Heiss WD. EEG power changes are related with regional cerebral glucose metbolism in vascular dementia. Clin Neurophysiol 1999;110:615–20.

Nunez, P.L., Wingeier, B.M., Silberstein, R.B., 2001. Spatial– temporal structures of human alpha rhythms: theory, microcurrent sources, multiscale measurements, and global binding of local networks. Hum. Brain Mapp. 13, 125–164.

Paré D, Collins DR, Pelletier JG (2002) Amygdala oscillations and the consolidation of emotional memories. *Trends Cogn Sci.* 6(7), 306-314.

Pariente J, Cole S, Henson R, Clare L, Kennedy A, Rossor m *et al.*, Alzheimer's patients engage an alternative network during a memory task. Ann Neurol 2005; 59: 870-879.

Petersen RC, Doody R, Kurz A, Mohs RC, Morris JC, Rabins PV, Ritchie K, Rossor M, Thal L, Winblad B (2001) Current concepts in mild cognitive impairment. *Arch Neurol* 58(12), 1985–92.

Petersen RC, Smith GE, Ivnik RJ, Tangalos EG, Schaid SN, Thibodeau SN, Kokmen E, Waring SC, Kurland LT (1995) Apolipoprotein E status as a predictor of the development of Alzheimer's disease in memoryimpaired individuals. *J Am Med Assoc* 273, 1274–8.

Petersen RC, Smith GE, Waring SC, Ivnik RJ, Kokmen E, Tangelos EG (1997) Aging, memory, and mild cognitive impairment. *Int Psychogeriatr*; 9 (Suppl. 1), 65–9.

Petersen RC, Smith GE, Waring SC, Ivnik RJ, Kokmen E, Tangelos EG. Aging, memory, and mild cognitive impairment. Int Psychogeriatr 1997;9(Suppl. 1):65–9.Petersen RC. Mild cognitive impairment: transition between aging and Alzheimer's disease. Neurologia. 2000 Mar;15(3):93-101.

Pijnenburg YAL, Made Y, Knol DL, van Cappellen van Walsum AM, Knol DL, Scheltens P, Stam CJ. EEG synchronization likelihood in midl cognitive impairment and Alzheimer's disease during a working memory task. Clin Neurophysiol 2004; 115: 1332-1339.

Portet F, Ousset P J, Visser P J, Frisoni G B, Nobili F, Scheltens Ph, Vellas B, Touchon J and the MCI Working Group of the European Consortium on Alzheimer's Disease (EADC, 2006) Mild cognitive impairment (MCI) in medical practice: a critical review of the concept and new diagnostic procedure. Report of the MCI Working Group of the

European Consortium on Alzheimer's Disease. *J Neurol Neurosurg Psychiatry* 77, 714-718.

Price JL, Morris JC. Tangles and plaques in nondemented aging and preclinical Alzheimer's disease. Ann Neurol 1999; 45: 358-368.

Radloff, LS (1977) The CES-D scale: A self-report depression scale for research in the general population. *Applied Psychological Measurement* 1, 385-401.

Rosen WG, Terry RD, Fuld PA, Katzman R, Peck A (1980) Pathological verification of ischemic score in differentiation of dementias. *Ann Neurol* 7(5), 486–8.

Rozzini L, Vicini Chilovi B, Conti M, Delrio I, Borroni B, Trabucchi M, Padovani A. Neuropsychiatric symptoms in amnestic and nonamnestic mild cognitive impairment. Dement Geriatr Cogn Disord. 2008;25(1):32-6.

Sauseng P, Klimesch W, Doppelmayr M, Hanslmayr S, Schabus M, Gruber WR. Theta coupling in the human electroencephalogram during a working memory task. Neurosci Lett 2004; 354:123–126.

Schonheit B, Zarski R, Ohm TG. Spatial and temporal relationships between plaques and tangles in Alzheimer pathology. Neurobiol Aging 2004; 25: 697-711.

Shulman KI: Clock-drawing: is it the ideal cognitive screening test? Int J Geriatr Psychiatry 2000; 15: 548–561.

Seidenbecher T, Laxmi TR, Stork O, Pape HC. Amygdalar and hippocampal theta rhythm synchronization during fear memory retrieval. Science 2003; 301:846–850.

Spinnler H, Tognoni G (1987) Standardizzazione e taratura italiana di test neuropsicologici. *Ital J Neurol Sci* 6 (suppl 8),1–120.

Stam C.J., van der Made Y., Pijnenburg Y.A., Scheltens P. EEG synchronization in mild cognitive impairment and Alzheimer's disease. Acta Neurol Scand 2003, 108: 90-96.

Steriade M, Llinas RR. The functional states of the thalamus and the associated neuronal interplay. Physiol Rev 1988;68:649–742.

Steriade M. Grouping of brain rhythms in corticothalamic systems. Neuroscience 2006; 137: 1087-1106.

Szelies B, Mielke R, Kessler J, Heiss WD. EEG power changes are related with regional cerebral glucose metbolism in vascular dementia. Clin Neurophysiol 1999;110: 615–20.

Tales A, Haworth J, Nelson S, Snowden RJ, Wilcock G. Abnormal visual search in mild cognitive impairment and Alzheimer's disease. Neurocase 2005a; 11: 80-84.

Tales A, Snowden RJ, Haworth J, Wilcock G. Abnormal spatial and non-spatial cueing effects in mild cognitive impairment and Alzheimer's disease. Neurocase. 2005b Feb;11(1):85-92.

Young KA, Holcomb LA, Bonkale WL, Hicks PB, Yazdani U, German DC. 5HTTLPR polymorphism and enlargement of the pulvinar: unlocking the backdoor to the limbic system. Biol Psychiatry. 2007 Mar 15;61(6):813-8.

Zalay OC, Bardakjian BL. Simulated mossy fiber associated feedforward circuit functioning as a highpass filter. Conf Proc IEEE Eng Med Biol Soc. 2006;1:4979-82.

Zappoli R, Versari A, Paganini M, Arnetoli G, Muscas GC, Gangemi PF, Arneodo MG, Poggiolini D, Zappoli F, Battaglia A. Brain electrical activity (quantitative EEG and bit-mapping neurocognitive CNV components), psychometrics and clinical findings in presenile subjects with initial mild cognitive decline or probable Alzheimer-type dementia. Ital J Neurol Sci 1995;16(6):341–76.

Zheng L., Jiang Z. Yu E. Alpha spectral power and coherence in the patients with mild cognitive impairment during a three-level working memory task. Journal of Zhejiang University SCIENCE B 2007; 8: 584-592.